KETO FOR WOMEN OVER 50:

The Complete Guide with 35-Day Meal Plan and 125 Recipes That Provenly Help To Drop Weight By Following The Ketogenic Diet Without Saying No To Delicious-Tasting Food

JULIANNE HALEY

Table of Contents

Introduction

In this book, you will find out why women who are over 50 will have to make some adjustments to the ketogenic diet. Since a woman's body goes through a lot of changes during that time, a different approach is needed. But don't worry, it's not that big a shift. I will also cover how you can slow down the aging process by eating less, but more nutritious food.

What Keto Does to a Woman's Body

We've already established that the ketogenic diet has various positive health benefits. But are there any advantages specific for women over 50? Although most of the research done on keto is based on the effects on men, a respectable number focused chiefly on women. The results indicate that keto is definitely a worthwhile diet for older women.

Helps Control Blood Glucose

Stable blood sugar levels are important. Excess insulin throws out essential hormones that regulate ovulation. Considering that insulin resistance, obesity, and type 2 diabetes often go hand in hand, getting your blood glucose levels under control and losing weight will get you one step closer to conceiving.

As we know, keto doesn't cause blood sugar spikes, which leads to weight gain and type 2 diabetes. In fact, studies done explicitly on women found that over four months, obese women with type 2 diabetes not only lost a lot of weight, but their fasting blood sugar and hemoglobin A1c (HbA1c) also improved markedly (Goday et al., 2016). The HbA1c count is a good indication of long-term blood glucose control.

Helps with Depression

A 2019 study found that the keto diet, in combination with psychotherapy and regular exercise, cured a 65-year-old woman's depression. She had had type 2 diabetes and clinical depression for 26 years, but as soon as she started eating low carb and her Hba1c dropped, she no longer had type 2 diabetes, and her depression was gone (Cox et al., 2019).

Reduces Inflammation in the Body

Inflammation is very dangerous; it harms cells in the body. Cardiovascular disease is only one of the many adverse effects of inflammation.

Less severe consequences include skin outbreaks, weight gain, lethargy, and body aches. A lot of women experience these daily because the carbohydrate consumption that is part of the standard American diet triggers inflammatory pathways. Since you won't be eating carbs on keto, inflammation is stopped in its tracks.

Relieves Symptoms of Menopause

As menopause draws near, estrogen levels drop. When this happens, women get hot flashes, battle depression, experience mood swings, and gain weight. But, when you eat keto, you will be consuming foods that increase estrogen, including broccoli and cauliflower, sesame seeds, flaxseeds, and walnuts.

Complements Cancer Treatment

Research has found that a ketogenic diet is beneficial to cancer patients (Branco et al., 2016). A study of 45 women who were diagnosed with endometrial or ovarian cancer found that keto decreased insulin-like growth factor (IGF-I) in the body. This hormone is claimed to encourage the spread of cancer (Cohen et al., 2018). Scientists believe the decrease of IGF-I and blood glucose creates an unreceptive environment for cancer cells.

Effective in Treating PCOS

Polycystic ovarian syndrome affects as many as 5 million American women of reproductive age. Still, the negative impact on health continues well into menopause and beyond (Centers for Disease Control and Prevention, n.d.). Since eating keto promotes weight loss—one of the primary factors in managing PCOS—hormone levels will return to normal, and for women who are still of child-bearing age, falling pregnant becomes more likely (McGrice & Porter, 2017).

Even though there are numerous health benefits to following the ketogenic diet, it may not be healthy for everyone.

Women who suffer from the following should not attempt to eat low carb without the guidance of a health professional:

- Liver of kidney failure
- Alcohol or drug abuse
- Type 1 diabetes
- Pancreatitis
- Disorders that affect fat metabolism Carnitine deficiency
- Additionally, women who are pregnant or breastfeeding should avoid eating keto.

The Gender and Age Difference

I mentioned earlier how not a lot of keto studies have been done on female subjects. There's still a lot we don't know. Yes, it is possible to reason that lower blood sugar levels and subsequent insulin regulation can prevent diabetes, but it still amounts to guesswork. That being said, the limited studies that have been done found there are significant differences between the two genders and how they react to keto. The main factor that contributes to these dissimilarities comes down to hormones.

Hormones and Keto

As a woman, you know that if your hormones are out of balance, then your life is too. Hormones are a fundamental part of every process in a woman's body, from reproduction to stress management. It doesn't

11

help that they tend to fluctuate during various times of the month, and due to other reasons, such as a lack of sleep.

Although men have hormones too, they're not nearly as sensitive to change. And keto is a pretty drastic change, so women have to pay extra attention to how they feel.

When you first switch over to eating low carb, the following may occur:

You may experience a lower sex drive, vaginal dryness, moodiness, and insomnia. This is due to low estrogen levels caused by cutting out processed foods containing soybean oil, which promote estrogen production, or due to menopause. If you want to raise your estrogen levels—which I recommend doing when you're over 50—eat more fat.

Keto may also increase the stress hormone cortisol. When your body realizes it doesn't have enough glucose in its system, it triggers a stress response and cortisol is released. This chronic stress may lead to an imbalance of blood glucose levels, decreased bone density, and a loss of muscle. But, considering that eating carbohydrates also causes fluctuating blood sugar levels, and a slew of other things, extra cortisol is not the worst that could happen.

The Menstrual Cycle

This is another thing woman have to face, and men don't. I know you may be thinking why include the menstrual cycle if this book is targeted at women 50 years and older. Well, late-onset menopause is a reality. Some women may continue to menstruate even after the age of 55 (AsiaOne, n.d.).

What makes periods extra difficult when you're following keto is the powerful cravings, which makes eating low carb particularly challenging.

Other than that, you feel bloated, and you're holding on to more water than usual—this reflects on the scale, which is in itself, discouraging. You get headaches, which may turn into a keto headache if you don't pay attention to your electrolyte balance and stay hydrated.

Digestion is an issue, and you more than likely feel like eating a bowl of pasta instead of meat and veggies packed with fiber. And then there are the cramps…

This is why so many women fall off the keto bandwagon at that time of the month—something men won't understand.

What Your Body Needs After 50

If you're 50, you're most likely in menopause or very close to it. As your hormone levels shift, your body changes. You won't be able to stop this process, but if you respond to these changes correctly, you may be able to slow it down!

Here are some changes you can expect when you hit the 50-year mark, and how you can use keto to give your body what it needs to stay healthy.

- *Your metabolism will slow down:* A slower metabolism means it will take fewer calories for you to gain weight. The high-fat aspect of keto curbs any hunger pangs, and you will automatically eat less to counter a sluggish metabolism.

- *Hormonal changes may cause digestive issues:* Cutting carbohydrates from your diet will promote a healthy gut, which will ease issues like irritable bowel disease or other inflammatory bowel issues.

- *Bone loss accelerates:* The drop in estrogen as you approach or enter menopause is to blame for a loss of bone density. Exercise will help but eating foods that raise your estrogen levels is also a good idea. The ketogenic diet contains a lot of these foods, among them kale and olives.

- *Your body stores more fat:* Fat, protein, and enough fiber will kill any cravings you have and will make it easier to avoid temptation. If you don't eat in excess, there won't be fat for your body to hold on to.

- *Your skin changes:* Bone broth is a great source of collagen, which helps your skin maintain its elasticity.

- *Your libido declines:* Removing sugary foods and carbs from your diet will help boost your sex drive.

- *Calcium deficiency becomes a reality:* The ketogenic diet allows you to eat dairy, but furthermore, kale, and broccoli, which are stapled low-carb veggies, are high in calcium.

A lot of what we experience as we grow older isn't pleasant, but it is in our power to not only make it more bearable but to slow the whole process down.

It's already evident that following a wholesome, nutritious diet will prolong your life by eliminating and preventing dangerous diseases. But calorie restriction also has the ability not only to increase your life but your lifespan. Here's how.

In one study, participants were asked to eat 15% fewer calories for two years. After the time elapsed, researchers found that not only were their metabolisms slower (meaning their bodies were more energy efficient), they also had less oxidative stress (Redman et al., 2018).

Cutting Calories Can Even Reduce Your Risk of Getting Age-Related Diseases

It all comes down to slowing your basal metabolism. According to Redman and associates, if a person's metabolism is slow, energy is spent more economically, which means cells and organs can 'work' less, and this increases their longevity. Although there are other factors, such as oxidative stress and dietary and biological elements that influence your metabolism, cutting calories is an excellent way to get it where healthy aging is possible.

Keto Challenges After 50

It's no wonder that your body will react adversely when you first start keto; cutting carbs from your diet basically turns everything upside down. It all of a sudden has to learn to use ketones as fuel instead of glucose. So, during this transition, you may not feel your greatest. Almost everyone who starts keto experiences some or all of these symptoms:

- Nausea
- Fatigue
- Headache
- Keto flu
- Irritability
- Lack of motivation

- Sugar cravings
- Brain fog
- Dizziness
- Keto rash
- Constipation
- Diarrhea

But, since you're a woman over 50, you may have to face some extra stumbling blocks, chiefly:

Your weight loss plateaus: If this happens, up to your fat consumption to the 80% mark.

Hormone imbalances: Don't restrict your calories too much and don't lose too much weight. A woman's body is healthiest with 22 to 29 percent body fat. Another way to combat these pesky hormones is to sync your diet with your menstrual cycle. When your period starts, eat more protein, then from days 6 to 11, go to the extreme end of low carb, and on days 12 to 16 eat a lot of avocados, broccoli, garlic, and parsley. You can end your cycle (days 17 to 28) by eating moderate low carb.

How Ketogenic Metabolism Works

Ketosis is a standard metabolic procedure that offers various wellbeing favorable circumstances.

During ketosis, your body changes over fat into mixes known as ketones and begins to utilize them as its essential wellspring of vitality.

Studies have found that consumes fewer calories that energize ketosis are very valuable for weight reduction owing to some degree to hunger suppressant impacts.

Rising examination shows that ketosis may likewise be valuable for, among different conditions, type 2 diabetes and neurological issue.

That being stated, accomplishing ketosis can set aside some effort to work and plan. It's not as simple as cutting carbs.

Here are some productive tips for getting into ketosis.

Reduce Your Carb Consumption

Expending a low-carb diet is by a wide margin the most critical factor in achieving ketosis.

Typically, your cells use glucose or sugar as their essential fuel source. In any case, the majority of your cells can likewise utilize different wellsprings of vitality. This includes unsaturated fats, just as ketones, which are otherwise called ketones.

Your body stores glucose in the liver and muscles as glycogen.

At the point when the utilization of starches is extremely little, the glycogen stores decline and the hormone insulin focuses decline. This empowers unsaturated fats to be discharged from your muscle versus fat's stores.

Your liver changes a bit of these unsaturated fats to ketone, beta-hydroxybutyrate, and acetoacetate. These ketones can be used as fuel for parts of the cerebrum.

The proportion of carb obstruction required to cause ketosis is somewhat individualized. A couple of individuals need to bind net carbs (complete carbs short fiber) to 20grams for consistently, while others can accomplish ketosis by eating twice so a great deal or more.

Subsequently, the Atkins diet confirms that carbs should be confined to 20 or fewer grams for consistently for around fourteen days to ensure that ketosis is cultivated.

After this stage, modest quantities of carbs can be familiar with your eating routine a little bit at a time, as long as ketosis is ensured. In one-week research, people with type 2 diabetes who had limited carb utilization to 2 1grams or less every day experienced day-by-day urinary ketone discharge rates that were multiple times more noteworthy than their standard fixations.

In another exploration, grown-ups with type 2 diabetes were allowed 20-50grams of edible carbs every day, in light of the number of grams that allowed blood ketone focuses on being kept up inside the objective scope of 0.5-3.0 mmol/L.

These carb and ketone ranges are prescribed for people who need to get ketosis to energize weight reduction, control glucose fixations, or lessening hazard factors for coronary illness.

Helpful ketogenic abstains from food utilized for epilepsy or exploratory disease treatment, then again, regularly limit carbs to under 5 percent of calories or under 15grams for each day to additionally build ketone levels.

Nonetheless, any individual who utilizes an eating regimen for restorative reasons should just do as such under the direction of a clinical expert.

Restricting your starch utilization to 20-50 net grams for every day lessens glucose and insulin fixations, prompting the arrival of putting away unsaturated fats that your liver proselytes to ketones.

Incorporate Coconut Oil in Your Diet

The utilization of coconut oil can help you to get into ketosis.

It includes fats called medium-chain triglycerides (MCTs).

In contrast to most fats, MCTs are immediately ingested and taken directly to the liver, where they can be utilized in a split second for vitality or changed to ketones.

As a general rule, it has been proposed that the utilization of coconut oil might be perhaps the most ideal approach to help ketone focuses on people with Alzheimer's ailment and different sensory system diseases.

Despite the fact that coconut oil incorporates four sorts of MCTs, half of its fat is gotten from the sort known as lauric corrosive.

A few examinations propose that fat sources with a more noteworthy extent of lauric corrosive may produce a progressively consistent measure of ketosis. This is on the grounds that it is more continuously used than different MCTs.

MCTs have been utilized to cause ketosis in epileptic children without restricting carbs as definitely as the exemplary ketogenic diet.

In actuality, a few preliminaries have found that a high-MCT diet including 20 percent of starch calories creates impacts tantamount to the great ketogenic diet, which offers under 5 percent of sugar calories.

While adding coconut oil to your eating routine, it's a smart thought to do so gradually to limit stomach related reactions, for example, stomach squeezing or loose bowels.

Start with one teaspoon daily and work up to a few tablespoons every day for seven days. You can find coconut oil in your neighborhood supermarket or get it on the web.

Devouring coconut oil offers your body with MCTs that are quickly retained and changed into ketone bodies by your liver.

Enhance Your Physical Activity

An expanding measure of examination has demonstrated that ketosis can be helpful for certain sorts of athletic execution, including continuance work out.

What's more, being progressively dynamic may help you get into ketosis.

At the point when you practice, your body will be drained from its glycogen shops. Typically, these are renewed when you expend carbs that are separated into glucose and afterward changed into glycogen.

In any case, if the utilization of sugar is limited, the glycogen stores remain little. In response, your liver improves the yield of ketones, which can be utilized as an elective wellspring of vitality for your body.

One examination found that activity improves the rate at which ketones are produced at low blood ketone levels. Be that as it may, when blood ketones are raised, they don't increment with practice and may viably diminish for a short timeframe.

Also, it has been demonstrated that turning out to be in a fasted state is driving up ketone focuses.

In a little examination, nine old females performed either preceding or after a supper. Their blood ketone focuses were 137-314 percent more prominent when utilized before a supper than when utilized after a dinner.

Remember that despite the fact that activity rises ketone yield, it might take one to about a month for your body to acclimate to the utilization of ketones and unsaturated fats as principle energizes. Physical execution might be diminished immediately during this second.

Taking part in physical activity may support ketone fixations during carb restriction. This effect can be improved by working in a quick paced state.

Ramp Up Your Healthy Fat Intake

A lot of good fat can expand your ketone focuses and assist you with accomplishing ketosis.

Indeed, an exceptionally ketogenic diet which is low carbs restricts carbs as well as high in fat.

Ketogenic eats less carbs for weight lessening, metabolic wellbeing and exercise proficiency by and large give between 60-80 percent of fat calories.

The classic ketogenic diet used for epilepsy is significantly more noteworthy in fat, with commonly 85-90 percent of calories in fat.

Be that as it may, incredibly raised fat utilization doesn't really bring about more prominent ketone focuses.

A three-week exploration of 11 sound individuals differentiated the effects of fasting with particular amounts of fat utilization on ketone centralizations of relaxing.

In general, ketone focuses have been found to be tantamount in people who expend 79% or 90% of fat calories.

Additionally, on the grounds that fat makes up such a major extent of the ketogenic diet, it is fundamental to pick top notch sources.

Extraordinary fats consolidate olive oil, avocado oil, coconut oil, spread, oil, and sulfur. Moreover, there are various strong, high-fat sustenance that are in like manner little in carbs.

Nevertheless, if your goal is weight decrease, it's fundamental to guarantee you don't exhaust such countless calories inside and out, as this can make your weight decrease delayed down.

Exhausting on any occasion 60 percent of fat calories will help increase your ketone centers. Pick the extent of sound fats from both animal and plant sources.

Try a Fat Fast or Short Fast

The other method to get into ketosis is to abandon eating for a couple of hours.

Actually, numerous people have gentle ketosis among lunch and breakfast.

Youngsters with epilepsy now and then fast for 24-48 hours before they start a ketogenic diet. This is accomplished to get into ketosis quickly with the goal that seizures can be diminished all the more quickly.

Irregular fasting, a wholesome technique including intermittent momentary fasting, may likewise cause ketosis.

Likewise, "fat fasting" is another ketone-boosting system that mirrors the effects of fasting.

It incorporates expending around 1,000 calories every day, 85-90 percent of which originate from fat. This blend of low calories and an extremely raised utilization of fat can help you accomplish ketosis quickly.

A 1965 exploration uncovered a significant loss of fat in overweight patients who followed a speedy fat. Be that as it may, different researchers have called attention to that these discoveries seem to have been incredibly misrepresented.

Since fat is so little in protein and calories, a limit of three to five days ought to be followed to evade an inordinate loss of bulk. It might likewise be difficult to adhere to for in excess of a couple of days.

Fasting, irregular fasting, and "fat fasting" would all be able to help you get into ketosis relatively quickly.

Maintaining Adequate Protein Intake

Showing up at ketosis needs a protein use that is fitting anyway not over the top.

The commendable ketogenic diet used in epilepsy patients is obliged to increasing ketone centers in both carbs and proteins.

A comparative eating routine may in like manner be important to infection patients as it would restrain tumor improvement.

In any case, it's definitely not a not too bad practice for the vast majority to decrease proteins to enable ketone to yield.

In any case, it is basic to eat up enough protein to effortlessly the liver with amino acids that can be used for gluconeogenesis, which means 'new glucose.' In this strategy, your liver offers glucose to a couple of cells and organs in your body that can't use ketones as fuel.

The Cornerstones of Ketogenic Diet

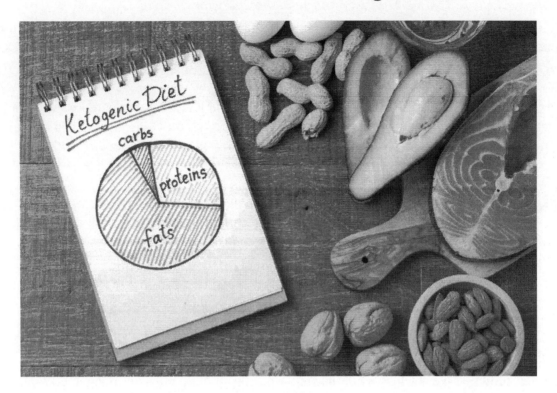

The ketogenic diet is a low-carb diet where you eliminate or minimize carbohydrates' consumption. Proteins and fats replace the extra carbs while you cut back on pastries and sugar.

How Does It Work?

See, when you consume less than 50g of carbs per day, your body starts to run out of blood sugar (which is used as fuel to provide your body quick energy). Once there are no sugar reserves left, your body will utilize fat and protein for energy. *This entire process is known as ketosis,* and this is exactly what helps you lose weight.

Compared to other diets, *Keto has a better chance of helping you lose weight more quickly.* The diet is also incredibly popular as you're not encouraged to starve yourself. It would help if you worked towards a more high-fat and protein diet, which isn't as difficult as counting calories.

Why Is It Important for People over 50?

Now comes the interesting part. I am sure you have been wondering how it will help you, a person who is 50 years or more in age, and why is it so important, right? Do not worry, as I shall provide you with an answer that satisfies both questions.

A few minutes ago, we read how the Keto diet pushes our body into ketosis, a state where *ketones take over glucose's role.* That may sound good for younger people than you, but the fact is that it is a better fit for someone your age. Why? I hear you ask.

As you grow in age, the body's natural fat-burning ability reduces. When that happens, your body stops receiving a healthy dose of nutrients properly, which is why you will develop diseases and ailments. With the Keto diet, you push the body into ketosis and bypass the need to worry about your body's ability to burn fat. *Once in ketosis, your body will now burn fat forcefully for survival.*

Once more, your system will now start to regain strength. An even better aspect that follows is your insulin level because it drops. If you are someone diagnosed with diseases such as type 2 diabetes and others, *the drop in insulin might even reverse the effects* and eliminate the diseases from your body altogether.

There are studies underway, and most of them suggest that the Keto diet is far more beneficial to those above 50 than it is for those under this age bracket. A quick search on *Google*® and you are immediately overwhelmed with *over 300 million results,* most of which explain the Keto diet's benefits for people above 50. That is a staggering number for a diet plan that has only been around a few years.

It is also important to highlight that as we get older, we start losing more than just the ability to burn fat. During this phase of our life, once we hit around 50 years of age, we come across various obstacles, some chronic in nature, which transpire only because our body can no longer function at rates like it did when we were young. *Ketogenic diets help us regain that edge and feel energized from within.*

There are hundreds of thousands of stories, all pointing out how this revolutionary diet is especially helpful for older adults and the elderly. Therefore, it is a no-brainer for people above 50 who have spent ages trying to search for a healthy lifestyle choice of diet. With such a high success rate, there is no harm in trying, right?

Before the Keto phenomenon, there was the *Atkins*® *diet.* The Atkins diet was also a low-carb diet, just like its Keto counterpart. This form of diet also became a huge hit with the masses. However, unlike Keto, the Atkins diet provided weight loss while putting a person through constant hunger. *Keto, on the other hand, takes away that element, and it does that using ketosis.*

Constant exposure to ketosis reduces appetite, hence taking away the biggest hurdle in most diets. The Atkins diet failed to address that front, which is why it was more of a hit and miss. However, credit where it is due, the Atkins diet did garner quite a bit of fame. However, since the inception of Keto, things have changed dramatically.

A study was conducted where 34 overweight adults were monitored and observed for 12 months. All of them were put on Keto diets. The result showed that participants had lower *HgbA1c* (hemoglobin A1C) levels, experienced significant weight loss, *and were more likely to discontinue their diabetes medications completely.*

All in all, the Keto diet is shaping up to be quite a promising candidate for older adults. Not only will this diet allow us to lead a healthier lifestyle, but it will also curb our ailments and ensure *high energy around the clock.* That is quite the resume for a diet and one that now seems too attractive to pass up. This is the point where I made up my mind and decided to give the Keto diet a go, and I recommend the same to you.

Whether you are a man or a woman, if you have put on weight or suffer from ailments like type 2 diabetes, consider this as your ticket to a care-free world where you will lead a healthy life and rise out of the ailments eventually.

Keto has been producing results that have attracted the top minds and researchers for a fairly long time. Considering the unique nature of this lifestyle of eating, the results have been rather encouraging.

"Great! How do I start?"

Not so fast. While the Keto diet is simple, I should point out a few things that you should know. Some of these might even change your mind about the entire Keto diet plan, but if you are determined for a healthy lifestyle and a fit body, I assure you these should not be of much trouble.

Preparing Yourself for Keto

When entering Keto's world, quite a few of us just pick up a recipe on the internet and start cooking things accordingly. While that is good, we tend to search for any specifics that we should know of, such as what would happen if I replace nuts with something else? Is oatmeal a part of the Keto diet? *What is Keto approved food item?* Are there any risks involved?

Here is some more information regarding such questions:

- Keto is an *extremely strict food diet* where you can only eat things that can be classified as Keto worthy. Anything that falls out of this category is a straight "no!"

- Keto is a completely new lifestyle. That means your body will undergo some changes. While most of these will be good, some may pose problems such as the *Keto flu.* Most of the people I know, including myself, faced this "flu" with similar influenza symptoms. It was only after some research that I realized this was natural. The Keto flu isn't exactly alarming, but it is best to be mentally prepared for it.

- You will need to work on your cooking skills as Keto strictly pushes processed, *high-carb foods out of the diet.*

- If you aren't really into the idea of protein and fat intake, you may wish to reconsider as these are the two primary areas Keto focuses on.

Apart from this, there are some mistakes people tend to make when they begin their journey. Some of the most common mistakes are:

- *Not knowing the Keto food properly:* Just because something looks like a Keto-friendly item doesn't mean it is Keto approved. Always refer to some food guide to check if the item you are interested in is a part of the "good food" in Keto.

- *Keeping the same level of fat intake throughout:* This often leads to results that show at the start and then disappear. You need to constantly adjust your diet and monitor your protein and fat intake.

- *Consuming bullet-proof coffee when you really shouldn't:* This coffee involves a mixture of coconut oil and butter within the coffee. While it is a perfect way to keep hunger at bay, it does push the level of bad cholesterol upwards. If you are someone who has been advised to stick to lower cholesterol levels and avoid consuming similar food items, keep this one off-limits.

- *Thinking the Keto flu is the only issue to face:* Other difficulties will emerge within the first ten weeks of your Keto journey. This will include lethargic limbs, which will make walking difficult at first. Owing to the change in fiber intake, you may either face diarrhea or constipation as well.

- *Pushing bodies with vigorous exercises:* You have just started Keto; give your body a bit of time to adjust. Keep things slow and steady.

- *Not replenishing on electrolytes:* Since we mentioned diarrhea and exercise, your body will run low on electrolytes faster than usual. This is something that you may want to keep in check. Think of sodium and potassium!

These are some of the most common mistakes people have made, and surprisingly, even I was no exception. If only I had someone to guide me back then properly.

Pathologies and Cases for which the Ketogenic Diet is not Recommended

While the ketogenic diet is suited for many different types of people, there are a few individuals who should avoid a low-carb, high-fat diet for a number of different reasons. Below, you will find a list of people who should not follow a ketogenic diet. If you see a condition you fall under; please visit your doctor or a professional who can select a diet better suited for you. Weight loss may be your ultimate goal, but your health always needs to come first.

Chron's Disease

If you have Chron's disease, this means that you have inflammation of the gut. Unfortunately, one of the major causes of gut inflammation is caused by animal products like meat and milk. While following the ketogenic diet, you will be on a high-meat diet and will be lacking the fibrous carbs that help promote gut health. When you limit carbohydrates, starches, and grains, this may worsen the symptoms of Chron's disease.

Cardiovascular Disease

As you may already know, animal products are high in cholesterol and high saturated fats. When they are consumed more often in a diet, this can clog arteries, which impacts the blood flow to the heart. The blood delivery is important to help get oxygen and nutrients to the rest of the cardiovascular system. The ketogenic diet is high in saturated animal fats and low in antioxidants that typically come from plant-sources. If you have a cardiovascular disease to begin with, this could increase the risk of developing further complications.

Chronic Fatigue Syndrome

As you first start out on the ketogenic diet, a high-fat amount can be hard to metabolize before your body makes the switch. Due to the fact that meat is harder to break down compared to plants in the digestive system, this can increase the amount of fatigue an individual feel. When you are eating a high-fat meal every day, all the time, this can put the digestive system into overdrive and make you feel even more tired.

Acne Issues and Other Skin Problems

On the ketogenic diet, you will not be eating as many vegetables as you are probably used to. Vegetables are high in vitamins A, C, and E, which help protect the skin against UV rays, prevent the appearance of skin wrinkles, and produce collagen to restore your skin. When you begin to follow a diet that is high in meat and low in fruit, you may experience more skin issues such as acne if not given the proper supplements. While it is preventable, it is something you will need to be mindful of when beginning the ketogenic diet.

Underweight/Anorexic

Individuals who are Anorexic or underweight should also consider avoiding the ketogenic diet. As you are already slightly aware, the ketogenic diet helps the body use stored fat as energy. When you are underweight or anorexic, the process is compromised by a lack of fat in the first place. When this happens, it could cause symptoms such as dizziness, fatigue, and brain fog. If you suffer from an eating disorder such as anorexia, be sure to consult with a nutritionist or a medical professional before making drastic changes to your diet.

High Blood Pressure

While the ketogenic diet can lower blood pressure, the first few weeks of starting the diet could pose as a threat to those who have high blood pressure when done incorrectly. As you begin the ketogenic diet, this does reduce the blood pressure, but if it is done too quickly, it can cause symptoms such as weakness and dizziness. If you have high blood pressure, you will want to consult with a professional to avoid any damage to your system by dropping your blood pressure too quickly. The ketogenic diet can help in the long run, but it is useless if you don't start out on the right foot.

Pregnancy

The ketogenic diet can be very beneficial if you are trying to get pregnant in the first place, but it is generally not recommended to continue the diet once you are pregnant. Eating a whole-food, including all fruits and vegetables, are vital when growing a child. A complete diet and exercise routine will be much more beneficial whole pregnant. This is also true for those who are breastfeeding. A small amount of carbohydrates will be vital during this period of time to keep up with energy levels.

What Happens to Our Bodies After the Age of 50?

First, let's explore how a woman's body reacts to aging. We will cover areas difficult for women and other individuals on the plan. Many women are entering menopause, but you need to understand the process as it has effects on all women:

- Weight loss uplands—or including weight gain—are a standard uncertain block for females on keto. One way to fight back is to incorporate more fat or try periods of intermittent fasting.

- Confining your calories and carbs too much on a keto diet can lead to out-of-balance hormones.

- Adjusting your eating habits along with your cycle can keep your keto lifestyle and hormones more in-sync.

- Women who had identified that their energy is wearisome must do carb cycling—"carb-up" at least one time or two times per week plus starchy vegetables.

- When emotional eating is upsetting your keto labors, breakdown habit loops by substituting your activities in small customs.

- Ditching a deprivation mindset can help you reframe the narrative around your diet, enabling you to stick with it.

The Issues Explained Further

Your Metabolism Slows Down

The main element to remember is you need to take in fewer calories.

Your Brain May Weaken

Your brain is much like a muscle and must be used, or it will become weak and shrink. Do new things in your life and step out of your comfort zone. It pushes your brain into an active mode when you switch things up. It could be as simple as going down a different path on the way home or changing the way you eat! Break the routine and try intermittent fasting to help slow the aging process.

Your Short-Term Memory Changes

Have you ever been around an individual who is over 50? If you are close with that person, you may notice some of the short-term memories will begin to fade, which can impact your daily routines. It's often displayed in the form of slowed reaction times and poor judgment.

Your Skin Changes

You will experience a lack of estrogen, which affects your skin, making it have the appearance of cellulite more prevalent and crepe-like. You can use a remedy on the intermittent fasting plan. Have a bit of bone broth or a dash of collagen powder to a cup of coffee or smoothie.

Your Hair & Nails Become Stressed

It's vital to increase your calcium intake because, like your skin, your hair and nails also change. You may notice your nails are brittle, and your hair has a bunch of split ends.

You'll Have More Dental Issues

By the age of 50, your tooth enamel erodes, creating an increase in dental issues. The issues may require increased care to eliminate tooth pain and unwanted cavities. It's vital to have regular dental exams and stop some of the woes after 50.

Your Eyesight May Deteriorate or Weaken

As you age, the darkness may be your worst enemy, which increases the issues involved with depth and distance perception. It's probably not to drive except during daylight hours. It's essential to take care of your eyesight and visit your optician regularly.

You Are More Susceptible to Injuries

You don't think about injuries at 50 because your mindset still thinks it's as agile now as it was at 21. Unfortunately, you're more likely to suffer from medical issues like carpal tunnel syndrome, tendinitis, and plantar fasciitis. It's recommended to take frequent breaks if you're at a work desk all day. Exercise is the key, so stretch your forearms or develop another inventive way to keep your muscles active to avoid so many repetitive movements.

Hormonal Changes May Prompt Digestive Issues

As hormones change, expect the menopause changes (on average) by 51. It's possible you will suffer from gas, bloating, and constipation.

Your Muscle Loss Accelerates

Your peak of muscle mass generally occurs at the age of 25. After 50, the loss of hormones, such as the growth hormone, is reduced. Make adequate sleeping a goal since that's when your hormones are released. opt for short intervals and weight training, working hard at short intervals, "hit it and quit it!".

Your Bone Loss Accelerates

The menopause time brings forth acceleration for three to five years, leading to bone fractures, many times brought on by a fall. Workout using your major muscle groups for some improvement of bone protection. Try working out a couple of times each week.

You Lose Flexibility

Don't try to do the splits as you did in your younger years. Your tendons and muscles lose their elasticity. Your spinal discs will also degenerate with age, raising your chances of injuries. You may need to use alternative healthcare as part of your health regimen. Consider chiropractic care, massage therapy, and stretching exercises.

Your Body Stores More Fat

Aging causes your body to store fat readily and reluctantly burns fat, especially if you are dehydrated or stressed. Estrogen dropping adds to the adverse effects of stress. It also deviates the fat from reproductive areas. Thus, you gain weight around the belly—losing your hourglass figure. The intermittent fasting methods will assist you by providing snacks and treats to enjoy using the ketogenic dieting methods. Provide extra fiber and protein to reduce your cravings and keep you satiated longer.

Lactose Intolerance Becomes an Issue

Milk is considered the #1 calcium supplier for strong and healthy bones. Aging can bring forth problems with women digesting milk properly as she ages. Intermittent fasting can add back some of the calcium by providing your diet with leafy greens, Greek yogurt, hard cheese, kefir, and tofu.

Your Fat Will Redistribute

During child-bearing years, the woman's body has fat allocated to her thighs and hips to support carrying a child. That changes during menopause as the body produces less estrogen; the fat collects in the tummy area, called 'menopause belly.'

You May Develop Foot Conditions

Some individuals will have deformities, including bunions and hammertoes, as a part of the aging process. In some cases, they are hereditary. Choose a good-fitting shoe that's not too tight to dissuade the worsening of the problem.

Your Feet Will Change Shape

It sounds crazy, but you may notice your feet become wider or longer during the aging process. According to Dr. Petkov, a podiatrist in New Jersey, "They can grow half a size in a decade." Your feet can also become flat since the ligaments and tendons lose their resilience. You will find that weight is a huge factor. It's essential to have someone measure your feet every few years to ensure that you are buying the right shoe size.

Your Body Synthesizes Protein Less Effectively

After 50, it's essential to consume adequate protein in your diet, or muscle loss may result. Strength training can improve the process, so it's vital to enjoy a high-protein meal about one or two hours after you have your workout.

You Are More Prone to Calcium Deficiency

Your bones are weakened when calcium is depleted. The lack of calcium can lead to bone pain and tenderness or osteoporosis. You should ingest 1200 mg. of calcium daily. Once again, intermittent fasting using cheese and yogurt are excellent remedies. Other calcium-rich foods include kidney beans, kale, broccoli, oranges, sesame seeds, edamame, and almonds.

You Might Develop Dry Mouth

With aging, the possibilities of diabetes, high blood pressure, arthritis, and Parkinson's, many individuals suffer from dry mouth brought on by many of the popular medications used to treat the ailment. Dry mouth can also lead to fungal infections of the throat, tongue, and other areas, including tooth decay and gum disease. Drink lots of water to stay hydrated, ensuring you floss regularly to remove plaque and food stuck in your teeth.

Your Libido Declines as You Go Through Menopause

Get plenty of sleep and opt for strength training a couple of times each week. You should also perform short interval training sessions once or twice weekly. Reducing the amount of sugar and alcohol (if you drink) you consume can boost your libido.

How Keto Diet Will Help to Live Easier After 50 and Feel Energetic

The keto diet has become so popular in recent years because of the success people have noticed. Not only have they lost weight, but scientific studies show that the keto diet can help you improve your health in many others. As when starting any new diet or exercise routine, there may seem to be some disadvantages so we will go over those for the keto diet. But most people agree that the benefits outweigh the change period!

Losing Weight

For most people, this is the foremost benefit of switching to keto! Their preceding diet method may have stalled for them or they were noticing weight creeping back on. With keto, studies have shown that people have been able to follow this diet and relay fewer hunger pangs and suppressed appetite while losing weight at the same time! You are minimizing your carbohydrate intake, which means fewer blood sugar spikes. Often, those fluctuations in blood sugar levels make you feel hungrier and more prone to snacking in between meals. Instead, by guiding the body towards ketosis, you are eating a more fulfilling diet of fat and protein and harnessing energy from ketone molecules instead of glucose. Studies show that low-carb diets are very effective in reducing visceral fat (the fat you commonly see around the abdomen that increases as you become obese). This reduces your risk of obesity and improves your health in the long run.

Reduce the Risk of Type 2 Diabetes

The problem with carbohydrates is how unstable they make blood sugar levels. This can be very dangerous for people who have diabetes or are pre-diabetic because of unstable blood sugar levels or family history. Keto is a great option because of the minimal intake of carbohydrates it requires. Instead, you are harnessing most of your calories from fat or protein which will not cause blood sugar spikes and ultimately less pressured on the pancreas to secrete insulin. Many studies have found that diabetes patients who followed the keto diet lost more weight and ultimately reduced their fasting glucose levels. This is monumental news for patients who have unstable blood sugar levels or are hoping to avoid or reduce their diabetes medication intake.

Improve Cardiovascular Risk Symptoms to Overall Lower Your Chances of Having Heart Disease

Most people assume that following keto that is so high in fat content has to increase your risk of coronary heart disease or heart attack. But the research proves otherwise! Research shows that switching to keto can lower your blood pressure, increase your HDL good cholesterol, and reduce your triglyceride fatty acid levels. That's because the fat you are consuming on keto is healthy and high-quality fats, so they reverse many unhealthy symptoms of heart disease. They boost your "good" HDL cholesterol numbers and decrease your "bad" LDL cholesterol numbers. It also decreases the level of triglyceride fatty acids in the bloodstream. A top level of these can lead to stroke, heart attack, or premature death. And what are the top levels of fatty acids linked to?

High Consumption of Carbohydrates

With the keto diet, you are drastically cutting your intake of carbohydrates to improve fatty acid levels and improve other risk factors. A 2018 study on the keto diet found that it can improve 22 out of 26 risk factors for cardiovascular heart disease! These factors can be very important to some people, especially those who have a history of heart disease in their family.

Increases the Body's Energy Levels

Let's briefly compare the difference between the glucose molecules synthesized from a high carbohydrates intake versus ketones produced on the keto diet. The liver makes ketones and uses fat molecules you already stored. This makes them much more energy-rich and a lasting source of fuel compared to glucose, a simple sugar molecule. These ketones can give you a burst of energy physically and mentally, allowing you to have greater focus, clarity, and attention to detail.

Decreases Inflammation in The Body

Inflammation on its own is a natural response by the body's immune system, but when it becomes uncontrollable, it can lead to an array of health problems; some severe, and some minor. The health concerns include acne, autoimmune conditions, arthritis, psoriasis, irritable bowel syndrome, and even acne and eczema. Often, removing sugars and carbohydrates from your diet can help patients of these diseases avoid flare-ups—and the delightful news is keto does just that! A 2008 research study found that keto decreased a blood marker linked to high inflammation in the body by nearly 40%. This is glorious news for people who may suffer from an inflammatory disease and want to change their diet to see improvement.

Increases Your Mental Functioning Level

Like we elaborated earlier, the energy-rich ketones can boost the body's physical and mental levels of alertness. Research has shown that keto is a much better energy source for the brain than simple sugar glucose molecules are. With nearly 75% of your diet coming from healthy fats, the brain's neural cells and mitochondria have a better source of energy to function at the highest level. Some studies have tested patients on the keto diet and found they had higher cognitive functioning, better memory recall, and were less susceptible to memory loss. The keto diet can even decrease the occurrence of migraines which can be very detrimental to patients.

Decreases risk of diseases like Alzheimer's, Parkinson's, and epilepsy. They created the keto diet in the 1920s to combat epilepsy in children. From there, research has found that keto can improve your cognitive functioning level and protect brain cells from injury or damage. This is very good to reduce the risk of neurodegenerative disease which begins in the brain because of neural cells mutating and functioning with damaged parts or lower than peak optimal functioning. Studies have found that the following keto can improve the mental functioning of patients who suffer from diseases like Alzheimer's or Parkinson's. These neurodegenerative diseases sadly have no cure, but the keto diet could improve symptoms as they progress. Researchers believe that it's because of cutting out carbs from your diet, which reduces the occurrence of blood sugar spikes that the body's neural cells have to keep adjusting to.

Keto can regulate hormones in women who have PCOS (polycystic ovary syndrome) and PMS (pre-menstrual syndrome). Women who have PCOS suffer from infertility, which can be very heartbreaking for young couples trying to start a family. There is no cure for this condition, but we believe it's related to many similar diabetic symptoms like obesity and a high level of insulin. This causes the body to produce more sex hormones which can lead to infertility. The keto diet has become a popular method that tries to regulate insulin and hormone levels and could increase a woman's chances of getting pregnant.

What Happens and What are the Changes in the Human Body with Pre-Menopause and Menopause

Perimenopause

Women can start experiencing hormonal changes related to menopause, years before their menopause begins. This stage is known as perimenopause, and the average age that women enter this stage is 46, but, of course, this depends on many factors and is different for every woman.

During this stage, periods become unpredictable and less frequent, and this lasts for about 5 years. This stage lasts 6 years and ends one year after the woman's last period.

Estrogen at this stage—Dips irregularly.

Menopause

Women enter menopause when they are around 51 or 52 years old. You know you are officially in menopause if one year has passed since the last period (if some other medical condition does not cause that, that is). Although the menopause symptoms, such as night sweats and hot flashes, begin in the perimenopause stage, during actual menopause, they are at its peak in the menopause stage.

Estrogen at this stage drops rapidly, causing noticeable changes such as bone loss and extreme hot flashes.

Post-Menopause

Post-menopause is the stage that occurs after menopause is considered over, which varies from woman to woman. Typically, post-menopause occurs during women's 50s. And while the menopause stage is officially finished, most of the symptoms will still be there.

Estrogen at this stage continues dropping, which causes natural changes in the body. That may cause women to continue experiencing menopause symptoms (although not so severe) such as hot flashes.

But why does it all happen? To understand better the natural changes in your body, think of the hormones as little messengers that travel through the bloodstream and bring a dose of regulation to chemical and physical functions in our bodies. For women in their 50s, the main culprit for the change in their bodies is the ovaries.

The ovaries produce hormones that regulate the reproductive system—estrogen and progesterone. The hormones that control these two hormones are the Follicle-Stimulating Hormone (FSL) and the Luteinizing hormone (LH). At this point, we are more concerned with the FSL hormone.

The FSL hormone is the messenger that sends an order of estrogen production and contributes to the release of eggs from the ovaries. When the woman reaches a certain age and enters perimenopause, her ovaries produce a decreased amount of estrogen because the ovaries have fewer eggs than during the reproductive years. But since the FSL messenger doesn't get the memo that the release order shouldn't be sent because there aren't that many eggs, this hormone gets increased. Trying to stimulate the production of estrogen, during these years, women have a higher level of the FSH hormone in their blood.

Peri-menopausal and menopausal women often describe sudden feelings of anxiety, or of being "overwhelmed," or of feeling tearful for no reason. Others report feelings of depression, and some experience rage, again, for no obvious reason.

Estrogen is linked with the production of serotonin, one of the neurotransmitters involved in the regulation of emotions and moods.

Low serotonin is associated with low mood and confusion, high serotonin with happiness, and an increased ability to learn and carry out complex tasks. During midway, it is calm. Too high serotonin levels affect in a state alike to sedation, and very low is associated with some debilitating psychiatric conditions. Regulation of serotonin is essential for our emotional health, and most types of medication used in the treatment of depression have the effect of maintaining levels of serotonin in the blood.

Estrogen slows down the rate at which serotonin is taken out of the bloodstream and also increases the sensitivity of the brain to serotonin by increasing the number of serotonin receptors on the brain cells.

During "perimenopause," the levels of estrogen may rise sharply and then drop.

When estrogen rises, so do serotonin levels. When it crashes, serotonin levels do the same. Women are familiar with the effects of these types of changes as they are responsible for the emotional changes many of them experience just before a period, as estrogen levels drop dramatically (albeit temporarily).

So, throughout the perimenopausal and menopausal stage, women may be experiencing the equivalent of random PMT.

Serotonin is not the only neurotransmitter involved in estrogen related mood swings. Estrogen also slows down the rate at which both dopamine and norepinephrine are absorbed. Low estrogen results in low levels of these neurotransmitters. Dopamine is involved in regulating mood, and our feelings of reward and pleasure. Low levels result in depressing moods.

On the other hand, very high levels of dopamine lead to feelings of aggression, irritability, impulsivity, and, ultimately, psychosis. High levels of estrogen may keep dopamine levels too high. This explains the feelings of anger and aggression that some women experience as part of PMT—estrogen levels are at their highest just before they plummet at the end of a cycle.

Norepinephrine regulates the fight and flight response to the threat, as well as alertness and energy, and at high levels produce feelings of stress and anxiety. Break it down too fast, and we are left without energy and the capacity to respond to stressful situations. If levels build-up, we may be overcome with anxiety. Estrogen regulates the levels of norepinephrine through the same mechanism as dopamine.

Consequently, throughout the perimenopause, the influence of altering estrogen levels on serotonin, dopamine, and norepinephrine can result in moods that fluctuate from depression to rage.

This is, of course, the extreme. Many of us will survive with occasional feelings of anxiety or depression, and some will barely notice a difference.

What Can We Do about Mood Swings?

- **Exercise**

Exercise is a great mood enhancer. Not only does it release endorphins, another group of neurotransmitters that give us a natural "high," but it also raises the levels of dopamine, norepinephrine, and serotonin. If your dipping estrogen levels are getting you down, exercise can help to redress the balance. Any form of exercise, a vigorous walk, or even climbing a flight of stairs, can help.

It may be the last thing you feel like doing when you are in a low mood, but it is the quickest way to correct your rebellious physiology. Most of us would not hesitate to take a pill, side effects, and all if it was going to make us feel better instantly. Exercise can do exactly that, and the side effects are all good.

If your mood has swung into an angry phase, the increased levels of serotonin brought about by exercise can calm you, and you can burn off the surplus energy of outrage.

Some people find it easier to take exercise in an organized form. You do not necessarily have to join a class. There are plenty of online courses, and YouTube is a great source of self-help videos. In another instance, attending a class and being involved may be precisely what you need—we are all diverse.

- **Diet**

Eat a healthy diet. Go easy on caffeine, sugar, and alcohol, all of which may have effects both directly on mood, and indirectly on the important mood-regulating neurotransmitters.

Eating a healthy diet, low in processed foods, artificial colorings, salt, and sugar, can improve your energy levels and your general state of health, which will put you in a better state to deal with mood swings.

Diet is also important in helping to control or reduce your weight. How does this help with mood? Low self-esteem tends to creep in with menopause, as a manifestation of low mood, but also as a symptom of our concerns about aging. Staving off the middle-age spread or flaking extra pounds can aid with this. As you lose weight, exercise, with all its mood-enhancing benefits, exercise, with all its mood-enhancing benefits, becomes easier.

How Ketogenic Diet Can Help Pre-Menopausal and Menopause Women

How the Ketogenic Diet Can Aid with the Signs and Symptoms of Ageing and Menopause

For aging women, menopause will bring severe changes and challenges, but the ketogenic diet can help you switch gears effortlessly to continue enjoying a healthy and happy life. Menopause can upset hormonal levels in women, which consequently affects brainpower and cognitive abilities. Furthermore, due to less production of estrogens and progesterone, your sex drive declines, and you suffer from sleep issues and mood problems. Let's have a look at how a ketogenic diet will help solve these side effects.

Enhanced Cognitive Functions

Usually, the hormone estrogen ensures the continuous flow of glucose into your brain. But after menopause, the estrogen levels begin to drop dramatically, so does the amount of glucose reach the brain. As a result, your functional brainpower will start to deteriorate. However, by following the keto diet for women over 50, the problem of glucose intake is circumvented. This results in enhanced cognitive functions and brain activity.

Hormonal Balance

Usually, women face major symptoms of menopause due to hormonal imbalances. The keto diet for women over 50 works by stabilizing these imbalances such as estrogen. This aids in experiencing fewer and bearable menopausal symptoms like hot flashes. The keto diet also balances blood sugar levels and insulin and helps in controlling insulin sensitivity.

Intensified Sex Drive

The keto diet surges the absorption of vitamin D, which is essential for enhancing sex drive. Vitamin D ensures stable levels of testosterone and other sex hormones that could become unstable due to low levels of testosterone.

Better Sleep

Glucose disturbs your blood sugar levels dramatically, which in turn leads to poor quality of sleep. Along with other menopausal symptoms, good sleep becomes a huge problem as you age. The keto diet for women over 50 not only balances blood glucose levels, but also stabilizes other hormones like cortisol, melatonin, and serotonin warranting an improved and better sleep.

Reduces Inflammation

Menopause can upsurge the inflammation levels by letting potential harmful invaders in our system, which result in uncomfortable and painful symptoms. Keto diet for women over 50 uses healthy anti-inflammatory fats to reduce inflammation and lower pain in your joints and bones.

Fuel Your Brain

Are you aware that your brain is composed of 60% fat or more? This infers that it needs a larger amount of fat to keep it functioning optimally. In other words, the ketones from the keto diet serve as the energy source that fuels your brain cells.

Nutrient Deficiencies

Aging women tend to have higher deficiencies in essential nutrients such as, iron deficiency which leads to brain fog and fatigue; Vitamin B12 deficiency, which lead to neurological conditions like dementia; Fats deficiency, that can lead to problems with cognition, skin, vision; and Vitamin D deficiency that not only causes cognitive impairment in older adults and increase the risk of heart disease but also contribute to the risk of developing cancer. On a keto diet, the high-quality proteins ensure adequate and excellent sources of these important nutrients.

Controlling Blood Sugar

Research has suggested a link between poor blood sugar levels and brain diseases such as Alzheimer's disease, Parkinson's Disease, or Dementia.

Some factors contributing to Alzheimer's disease may include:

- Enormous intake of carbohydrates, especially from fructose - which is drastically reduced in the ketogenic diet.

- Lack of nutritional fats and good cholesterol - which are copious and healthy in the keto diet

Keto diet helps control blood sugar and improve nutrition, which in turn not only improves insulin response and resistance but also protects against memory loss which is often a part of aging.

Is it Possible to Have a Perfect Body even at 50?

How Does the Keto Diet Aid in Weight Loss?

With everything, how will the keto weight loss plan actually aid your body drop extra pounds? When on an excessive carb food plan, your frame uses glucose from carbohydrates then sugars to gas frame events. Once on a ketogenic eating routine, you stock the structure with minimum quantities of carbs and sugars.

With decreased sugar and carbs deliver, the glucose levels in the frame are depleted, inflicting the body to look for alternative strength resources. The body, consequently, goes to deposited fats for strength; that is the reason the Keto diet ends in weight loss.

This situation wherein your frame burns fat for strength apart from carbs is called ketosis. While your body is experiencing ketosis, it formed ketones as the gasoline source instead of relying on glucose. Ketones and glucose are the only two energy resources that feed the brain.

Benefits of Ketosis and the Keto Weight-Reduction Plan

Besides merely helping in weight reduction, setting the frame in ketosis comes with different health advantages too. Here are some of them:

- Enhanced mental clarity
- Improved physical power
- Steady blood sugar levels which make it an excellent remedy for epilepsy and diabetes
- Improved and enhanced skin tones
- Lower cholesterol stages
- Hormone law specifically in women

The Ketogenic eating regimen is one of the best diets you could observe for weight reduction and enhance your overall health. The diet also can be used for youngsters who are overweight. Numerous studies guide the weight-reduction plan showing good-sized results; you may find them online.

Keto food plan adherents, particularly the ones elderly 50 and older, are said to enjoy several capability health benefits including:

Increased Physical and Mental Energy

As humans develop older, energy levels would possibly drop for plenty of organic and environmental reasons. Keto eating regimen adherents frequently witness a lift in vitality and strength. One aim said incidence takes place is since the frame is burning excess fats, which in turn gets synthesized into electricity. Besides, complete synthesis of ketones will be predisposed to upsurge brain supremacy besides rouse cognitive roles like memory and focus.

Improved Sleep

Individuals generally tend to sleep much less as they age. Keto WeightWatchers frequently gain additional from exercising applications and grow to be worn-out easier. Said occurrence should precipitate longer and extra fruitful intervals of rest.

Metabolism

Aging individuals often experience a sluggish metabolism than they have for the duration of their more youthful days. Long-time keto WeightWatchers enjoy a more significant law of blood sugar, which can grow their metabolic rates.

Weight Loss

Extra green and faster metabolism of fats help the body remove accumulated body fats, which can precipitate the loss of excess pounds. Additionally, adherents also are believed to enjoy a concentrated appetite, which may cause a reduced caloric consumption.

Keeping the load off is crucial, particularly as adults age when they may need much fewer calories daily compared to while focusing in their 20s or 30s. Thus far it is miles still crucial to contract nutrient-wealthy food from this weight loss program for adults.

Since it is common for growing older adults to lose muscle and electricity, an excessive protein precise ketogenic food regimen can be endorsed via a nutritionist.

Protection Against Some Illnesses

Keto WeightWatchers over age 50 may want to lessen their risk of evolving illnesses inclusive of diabetes, mental problems like Alzheimer's, various cardiovascular maladies, multiple styles of cancer, Parkinson's Disease, Non-Alcoholic Fatty Liver Disease (NAFLD), and a couple of sclerosis.

Aging

Aging is taken into consideration by some as the most crucial danger issue for human ailments or disease. So, decreasing growing older is the logical step to minimize these dangerous elements of illness.

Right information extending from the technical description of the ketosis manner offered earlier, suggests the increased strength of teenagers as a result, and because of the utilization of fat as a fuel source, the body can undergo a procedure in which it may misunderstand signs so as to the mTOR signal is bottled-up and a loss of glucose is evident whereby it's far reported growing older may be slowed.

Generally, for years, more than one study has noted that caloric limit can resource to slowing growing old and even increase lifespan. With the ketogenic eating regimen, it's miles possible without decreasing calories to affect anti-growing old. An intermittent fasting method used with the keto weight loss plan also can have an impact on vascular aging.

If an individual fasts intermittently or when at the keto eating regimen, Beta-Hydroxybutyrate or BHB is produced that is supposed to result in anti-getting older effects.

How Does Women Initiate a Keto Diet?

Slowly and carefully. A ketogenic weight loss program should not be commenced at a complete a hundred percent. You have to lower the number of carbs you consume slowly. Cutting the carbs too quickly can have a negative effect. It can stress the frame and confuse it, therefore inflicting a wild imbalance.

Also, if pregnant or nursing, you have not to use a keto diet. During this period, eat a well-rounded weight loss program of fruits, vegetables, dairy, and grains.

My quality advice, get your body as healthy as possible, and then slowly contain a ketogenic weight loss program.

Advice on How to Best Follow the Keto Lifestyle

Some of them are relatively simple, while others will help you see things in a new and helpful way. You already know that the essential part of Keto is limiting your carb intake, but that doesn't make it easy to do in practice. Here is a list of tips that will make it easy.

Our first tip is about shopping for food. If you go grocery shopping with a predetermined list of items based on our 30-day diet plan, you won't even feel the need to buy anything that might contain carbs. You already know that you're buying good foods that stay within the confines of Keto, so it won't even cross your mind.

This tip goes with the most important advice I have for you, which is not to overwhelm yourself.

Overwhelming yourself with all the possibilities of Keto is easy to do. The best way to avoid this is to know the ingredients you need for your meals before you cook them.

You already have a list of 30 meals that all follow the Keto diet's requirements. What comes next is being ready to cook these meals every day. Getting the ingredients in your pantry or fridge is the first thing you need to do.

You don't want to plan to eat the Keto taco casserole the next day and find out you are missing ground beef the day of. You can avoid making this mistake by looking at the ingredient lists ahead of time. Double-check it to make sure you have everything you need ahead of time.

But you might find that keeping track of every ingredient ahead of time is unrealistic. Luckily, there is an easier way to look at these ingredients. You can break down the ingredients you need into three groups: proteins, vegetables, and healthy fats.

The first one is the easiest to find. Be sure you always have protein sources in your home such as turkey, fish, pork, beef, and so on.

When you check your kitchen for vegetables, you want to stick with vegetables that are low in carbs, of course. Examples of vegetables that fit into this category include broccoli, cauliflower, cucumbers, and bell peppers.

Finally, you want to have fats in your diet, but they need to be healthy fats. If you don't know the difference, here is a quick run-down.

We have three basic kinds of fats: from least healthy to healthiest, we have trans fats, saturated fats, and unsaturated fats.

You never want to eat trans fats. In fact, they are even banned in the United States and many other countries. Saturated fats are not good for you, either, but you don't need to be concerned about getting a few grams of saturated fats here and there.

However, you want most of your fats to be unsaturated fats. Unsaturated fats fall into two categories that you will see on nutrition labels: polyunsaturated and monounsaturated fats. Be on the lookout for these, because they are the kinds of fats you want when you are on the Keto diet.

As long as you get unsaturated fats, proteins, and low-carb vegetables into your diet, you are on Keto. The 30 days of recipes will be of great help to you, but you don't need to follow them exactly. You will still be doing Keto if you follow these basic guidelines.

My next tip is to make it impossible to betray your new Keto diet. Women new to the diet often can't get started with it simply because they keep the same food in their house. It is certainly harder to change your diet when all the old foods you used to eat are lying around.

We say to ourselves that we don't want to waste food. Not wanting to waste food is a good virtue, but in practice, it only keeps us from changing our eating habits. We tell ourselves that we can change our habits later, but later never comes.

The only way to keep yourself from making this mistake is to get rid of the risk entirely. As long as you still have high-carb foods in your pantry and refrigerator, there is a very good chance you will still eat them.

I don't like to waste food either, so when I started Keto, I gave these foods to my parents. That way, the food didn't go to waste, but I didn't have to eat it and mess up my Keto routine.

Since you are new to Keto, you might not know what exactly you should get rid of. Now, you still have to make choices every day not to break with Keto. This tip will not keep you from ever "cheating" on Keto—but it will make it a whole lot easier if you give away all these items in your kitchen:

- Grains such as pasta, wheat, bread, rice, and cereal.
- Sweets—anything manufactured to be filled with sugar. This means candy, honey, soda, juice, syrup, chocolate, and cake.
- Potatoes and other starchy vegetables
- Legumes such as beans
- Fruits like oranges, grapes, apples, and bananas that are high in sugar
- Dairy products (they can be consumed in moderation, but you need to seriously limit your consumption of them)
- Processed foods in general. If you have any foods in your kitchen that are less than fresh, you will know what they are. Take these out of your kitchen.

When you rid your kitchen of these foods, you need foods to replace them with. Here is a place to start:

- Butter and coconut oil for their unsaturated fats
- Green vegetables such as kale, spinach, and lettuce
- Any vegetables low in carbohydrates such as cauliflower, asparagus, and zucchini
- Beef, pork, chicken, turkey, fish—any meat really, as long as you get them from a grocery store whose meat sources are grass-fed
- Lots of eggs

My next tip is to know the Keto staples.

In case you don't already know, Keto staples are foods that Keto practitioners eat every single day. Like all Keto foods, they are low-carb and often high in unsaturated fats. These foods are also easy to eat and usually are consumed in the form of snacks. Start replacing high-carb, heavily processed snacks with these Keto staples:

- Seeds and nuts like sunflower seeds, almonds, cashews, and peanuts in small amounts
- Flour substitutes such as coconuts flour and almond flour
- Sweet but sugarless drinks like black coffee and tea. Find a source of sweetening that has no sugar if you don't want to consume them plain
- By the same token, find a sugarless sweetener to give your water some taste

I can't overstate the importance of finding a sugar-free source of sweetener. People who can't stick with Keto sometimes have issues doing so because they feel like they can't get enough flavor while on the diet.

As you know from the 30-day Keto meal plan, this is not true—you can get all kinds of flavors while still on the diet.

The real problem is that people these days have a sugar addiction. We are so used to eating sugar all the time that we feel like we need it. We could criticize ourselves endlessly for being used to eating sweet food, but that wouldn't get us anywhere.

What we really need is a solution to this addiction to sweetness. Since we can't consume too much sugar on Keto, our best option is to replace it with sugarless sweeteners.

Now that we have spent plenty of time helping you to change the foods you eat; we are getting into the psychological side of changing your diet. This next tip is simple: take it easy.

There is a lot of incentive not to jump into Keto without caution. The Keto flu may be only temporary, but it tends to discourage women from continuing to do Keto, so it is still something worth avoiding. You are better off taking things slowly, so you don't shake the balance of your body's chemicals too much.

But how do you actually take it slowly? If you take Keto slowly, where do you start?

The trick to taking Keto slowly is to introduce one new lifestyle change at a time. For example, you could first try taking out all the sugar-filled foods in your kitchen, but don't do anything else. Just see how well you can get by without these foods.

Once you get used to your life without these foods, try to do something else, like eating more vegetables such as broccoli, cauliflower, and spinach. You might be hesitant to take Keto one thing at a time because you want to get the most possible health effect from it as quickly as possible.

However, the risk of burning out of Keto is real. That's why I suggest you make one small change towards Keto at a time—it is much more sustainable in the long term.

In the same vein, pay attention to the signs your body is giving you. You will be able to tell whether you are taking things too quickly or not.

A lot of people go wrong in this area because they get busy with day-to-day life and stop listening to their bodies.

Don't let this happen to you. Allow some time to yourself every day where you aren't consuming any media, whether it is music, TV, or the Internet. Do nothing but spend a little bit of time in silence every day.

It doesn't have to be more than five to ten minutes every hour. After that, you can go back to whatever it is you were doing. But especially when you are making such a drastic change to your body, you can't implement all these changes without listening to your body's response to it. Be sure you are ready for your body to tell you what to do next.

Another aspect of improving at listening to your body is realizing how slow your body is to tell you things. A good example of this is how long it takes for it to tell you that you are full.

All of us have experienced this. We finish our dinner, but afterwards, we still feel hungry. Then, we feel justified in continuing to eat because we think our bodies are telling us to keep eating. Even if we know logically that we shouldn't eat anymore, we look for any excuse to just do whatever it is we want to do.

There is a way to deal with this problem.

If you know that you have eaten plenty, but your body is telling you to eat more, find something else to get your mind occupied with for a while. You might still feel hungry after this time, and if so, you should be fine to eat.

That might mean your body really did need more energy. But more likely than not, your body was telling you to eat more because you were bored—or just because it tastes good. People easily confuse genuine hunger with mere craving. You can entertain yourself in ways other than eating so as to avoid this confusion.

My last tip for succeeding in Keto is to know how to approach these three nutrients: carbs, proteins, and healthy fats.

For carbs, you could know nothing more than not to eat more than 30grams of carbs every day. For protein, try to get 0.9grams of protein for every pound you weigh. Finally, for fats, try to reach 100grams of healthy fats every day.

Don't buy into the old paradigm that fats are bad. Fats are not the enemy—the enemy is eating too many calories without burning them off with exercise. Keeping carbs off is the best way to stay away from these extra calories in the first place.

What Side Effects the Ketogenic Diet Must Have

Low Energy Levels

When available, the body prefers to use carbohydrates for fuel as they burn more effectively than fats. General drop-in energy level is a concern raised by many dieters due to the lack of carbohydrates. Studies have shown that it causes orthostatic hypotension which causes lightheadedness. It has come to be known that these effects can be avoided by providing enough supplemental nutrients like sodium. Many of the symptoms can be prevented by providing 5grams of sodium per day. Most times, fatigue disappears after a few weeks or even days, if fatigue doesn't disappear, then you should add a small number of carbohydrates to the diet as long as ketosis is maintained. The diet is not recommended when caring out high-intensity workouts, weight training, or high-intensity aerobic exercise as carbohydrates are an absolute requirement but are okay for low-intensity exercise.

Effects on the Brain

It causes increased use of ketones by the brain. The increased use of ketones, among other reasons, result in the treating of childhood epilepsy. As a result of the changes that occur, the concern over the side effects, including permanent brain damage and short-term memory loss, has been raised. The origin of these concerns is difficult to understand. The brain is powered by ketones in the absence of glucose. Ketones are normal energy sources and not toxic as the brain creates enzymes, during fetal growth, that helps us use them. Epileptic children, though not the perfect examples, show some insight into the effects of the diet on the brain in the long term.

There is no negative effect in terms of cognitive function. There is no assurance that the diet cannot have long-term dietary effects, but no information proves that there are any negative effects. Some people feel they can concentrate more when on the ketogenic diet, while others feel nothing but fatigue. This is a result of differences in individual physiology. There are very few studies that vaguely address the point on short-term memory loss. This wore off with the continuation of the study.

Kidney Stones and Kidney Damage

As a result of the amplified job from getting to filter urea, ketones, and ammonia, as well as dehydration concerns of the potential for kidney damage or passing kidney stones have been raised. The rich nature of protein in the ketogenic diet raises the alarms of persons who are worried about possible kidney damage. There is very little information that points to any negative effects of the diet on kidney function or the development of kidney stones. There is a low incidence of small kidney stones in epileptic children, this may be as a result of the state of deliberate dehydration that the children are put at instead of the ketosis state itself.

Some short-term research shows no change in kidney function or increased incidents of kidney stones either after they are off the diet or after six months on a diet. There is no long-term data on the effects of ketosis on kidney function; thus, no complete conclusions can be made. People with preexisting kidney issues are the only ones who get problems from high protein intake. From an unscientific point of view, one would expect increased incidents of this to happen to athletes who consume very high protein diets, but it has not happened. This suggests that high protein intake, under normal conditions, is not harmful to the kidneys. To limit the possibility of kidney stones, it is advised to drink a lot of water to maintain hydration. People who are predisposed to kidney stones should have their kidney function monitored to ensure that no complications arise if they decide to follow through with the diet.

Constipation

A common side effect of the diet is reduced bowel activities and stultification. This arises from two diverse reasons: lack of fiber and gastrointestinal engagement of foods. Initially, the absence of carbs in the diet means that unless supplements are taken, fiber intake is low. Fiber is very important to our systems. High fiber intake can prevent some health conditions, including heart disease and some forms of cancer. Use some type of sugar-free fiber supplement to prevent any health problems and help you maintain regular bowel movements. The diet also reduces the volume of stool due to enhanced absorption and digestion of food; thus, fewer waste products are generated.

Fat Regain

Dieting, in general, has very low long-term success rates. There are some effects of getting out of a ketogenic diet like the regain of fat lost through calorific restriction alone. This is true for any diet based on calorific restrictions. It is expected for weight to be regained after carb reintroduction. For people who use the weighing scale to measure their success, they may completely shun carbs as they think it is the main reason for the weight regain. You should understand that most of the initial weight gain is water and glycogen.

Immune System

There is a large variety in the immunity system response to ketogenic diets on different people. There has been some repost on reduction on some ailments such allergies and increased minor sickness susceptibility.

Optic Neuropathy

This is optic nerve dysfunction. It has appeared in a few cases, but it is still existence. It was linked to the people not getting adequate amounts of calcium or vitamins supplements for about a year. All the cases were corrected by supplementation of adequate vitamin B, especially thiamine.

Mistakes Made on the Keto Diet and How to Overcome Them

Do you feel like you are giving your all to the keto diet, but you still aren't seeing the results you want? You are measuring ketones, working out, and counting your macros, but you still aren't losing the weight you want. Here are the most common mistakes that most people make when beginning the keto diet.

Too Many Snacks

There are many snacks you can enjoy while following the keto diet, like nuts, avocado, seeds, and cheese. But snacking can be an easy way to get too many calories into the diet while giving your body an easy fuel source besides stored fat. Snacks need to be only used if you frequently hunger between meals. If you aren't extremely hungry, let your body turn to your stored fat for its fuel between meals instead of dietary fat.

Not Consuming Enough Fat

The ketogenic diet isn't all about low carbs. It's also about high fats. You need to be getting about 75 percent of your calories from healthy fats, five percent from carbs, and 20 percent from protein. Fat makes you feel fuller longer, so if you eat the correct amount, you will minimize your carb cravings, and this will help you stay in ketosis. This will help your body burn fat faster.

Consuming Excessive Calories

You may hear people say you can eat what you want on the keto diet as long as it is high in fat. Even though we want that to be true, it is very misleading. Healthy fats need to make up the biggest part of your diet. If you eat more calories than what you are burning, you will gain weight, no matter what you eat because these excess calories get stored as fat. An average adult only needs about 2,000 calories each day, but this will vary based on many factors like activity level, height, and gender.

Consuming a lot of Dairies

For many people, dairy can cause inflammation and keeps them from losing weight. Dairy is a combo food meaning it has carbs, protein, and fats. If you eat a lot of cheese as a snack for the fat content, you are also getting a dose of carbs and protein with that fat. Many people can tolerate dairy, but moderation is the key. Stick with no more than one to two ounces of cheese or cream at each meal. Remember to factor in the protein content.

Consuming a lot of Protein

The biggest mistake that most people make when just beginning the keto diet is consuming too much protein. Excess protein gets converted into glucose in the body called gluconeogenesis. This is a natural process where the body converts the energy from fats and proteins into glucose when glucose isn't available. When following a ketogenic diet, gluconeogenesis happens at different rates to keep body function. Our bodies don't need a lot of carbs, but we do need glucose. You can eat absolute zero carbs, and through gluconeogenesis, your body will convert other substances into glucose to be used as fuel. This is why carbs only make up five percent of your macros. Some parts of our bodies need carbs to survive, like kidneys, medulla, and red blood cells. With gluconeogenesis, our bodies make and stores extra glucose as glycogen just in case supplies become too low.

In a normal diet, when carbs are always available, gluconeogenesis happens slowly because the need for glucose is extremely low. Our body runs on glucose and will store excess protein and carbs as fat.

It does take time for our bodies to switch from using glucose to burning fats. Once you are in ketosis, your body will use fat as the main fuel source and will start to store excess protein as glycogen.

Not Getting Enough Water

Water is crucial for your body. Water is needed for all your body does, and this includes burning fat. If you don't drink enough water, it can cause your metabolism to slow down, and this can halt your weight loss. Drinking 64 ounces or one-half gallon every day will help your body burn fat, flush out toxins, and circulate nutrients. When you are just beginning the keto diet, you might need to drink more water since your body will begin to get rid of body fat by flushing it out through urine.

Consuming Too Many Sweets

Some people might indulge in keto brownies and keto cookies that are full of sugar substitutes just because their net carb content is low, but you have to remember that you are still eating calories. Eating sweets might increase your carb cravings. Keto sweets are great on occasion; they don't need to be a staple in the diet.

Not Getting Enough Sleep

Getting plenty of sleep is needed in order to lose weight effectively. Without the right amount of sleep, your body will feel stressed, and this could result in your metabolism slowing down. It might cause it to store fat instead of burning fat. When you feel tired, you are more tempted to drink more lattes for energy, eat a snack to give you an extra boost, or order takeout rather than cooking a healthy meal. Try to get between seven and nine hours of sleep each night. Understand that your body uses that time to burn fat without you even lifting a finger.

Low on Electrolytes

Most people will experience the keto flu when you begin this diet. This happens for two reasons when your body changes from burning carbs to burning fat, your brain might not have enough energy, and this, in turn, can cause grogginess, headaches, and nausea. You could be dehydrated, and your electrolytes might be low since the keto diet causes you to urinate often.

Getting the keto flu is a great sign that you are heading in the right direction. You can lessen these symptoms by drinking more water or taking supplements that will balance your electrolytes.

Consuming Hidden Carbs

Many foods look like they are low carb, but they aren't. You can find carbs in salad dressings, sauces, and condiments. Be sure to check nutrition labels before you try new foods to make sure it doesn't have any hidden sugar or carbs. It just takes a few seconds to skim the label, and it might be the difference between whether or not you'll lose weight.

If you have successfully ruled out all of the above, but you still aren't losing weight, you might need to talk with your doctor to make sure you don't have any health problems that could be preventing your weight loss. This can be frustrating, but stick with it, stay positive, and stay in the game. When the keto diet is done correctly, it is one of the best ways to lose weight.

How Long Should Ketogenic Diet Last

I will cover the tweaks you can make to your Keto diet and lifestyle to accommodate these particular hurdles. I will address any concerns you may have and give you solutions to counteract them.

Women go through menopause sometime between the ages of 45 and 55, and it can be a particularly difficult time.

But many of these symptoms are temporary. The one that bothers women the most is the one that lasts: weight gain. Women over 50 want to know how they can stave off weight gain and lose the extra pounds they started to put on after menopause.

First of all, I highly recommend intermittent fasting for women in this age group. Intermittent fasting is often paired with Keto for the best possible results in autophagy. Autophagy can be improved through Keto alone, but you don't truly unlock the potential advanced autophagy in your body until you fast between your Ketogenic meals.

The reason I urge you to do intermittent fasting with Keto is that it will help you more with the effects of aging than Keto alone. The autophagy that results from fasting doesn't only help you get better skin, lose weight, and detox your cells—although all these things are worth trying to achieve on their own.

The long-term, anti-aging benefits of intermittent fasting are more important but often ignored. The autophagy that comes from intermittent fasting will help you lower your inflammation, boost your metabolism, enhance your immune system, and more. These are all benefits of autophagy that are backed by scientific research.

Studies show time and time again that fasting works to help women lose weight and improve their health. As a woman over 50, you should consider doing Keto together with fasting.

Scientists are not in agreement about whether menopause itself affects weight. Some say that when women gain weight at this stage in life, it is because of aging alone. They do not believe the hormonal changes from menopause are the reason for the weight gain.

But there is no denying that the lowered estrogen from menopause has some impact on the distribution of fat on the body of a woman over 50. You may have noticed this yourself in your own body: the change in hormones tends to make a woman's fat go from her hips to her waist.

That isn't all, either. Women who go through menopause also report that they have less energy and have a harder time burning fat. It is no wonder women over 50 want to know how to lose weight. It is such a harder feat at this stage in life.

But don't be misled to believe the change in metabolism is all that is going on here. After all, a doctor studying woman over 50 found that women's bodies only metabolized 50 calories fewer calories every day. While this is not a negligible figure, it can hardly be blamed for all of the weight gain that is experienced by women at this age.

You are sure to have experienced some of the other factors that play into weight gain for women at this age. Women over 50 report having more cravings, doing less exercise, and losing more muscle.

As you might guess, many of these factors are related. When you aren't exercising as much, you won't retain as much muscle. If you have more cravings for foods you shouldn't eat, you are more likely to eat those foods and gain weight as a result.

Top it all off with the less efficient metabolisms of women over 50, and it is easy to understand why they have a hard time losing weight. Even if menopause itself isn't the reason women experience this, it all adds up to make weight loss seem impossible, if you don't know anything about Keto or fasting.

Take everything you hear them say about weight gain for women over 50 with a grain of salt. All of us know that it is a reality for women who fall into this age range, but no one knows exactly what the reason for it is. But we do know that Keto and fasting both show fantastic results for these women, so that is the information we should really be paying attention to.

Women in this age range can still go wrong when they try Keto and autophagy, so I have some pieces of advice to give you if you count yourself among this group.

The first piece of advice is to make sure you eat enough protein every day. You might be worried about eating too much protein because you are watching calories, and this is a reasonable thing to do. But when you are on Keto, you need protein as a source of energy.

It is always about balance. On the one hand, you need to make up for the energy you won't be getting from carbs. On the other hand, you have to be careful not to eat too many calories.

As usual, follow along with what your body is telling you. If your body tells you that you still need more energy, wait a bit. You can eat more if some time passes and you still feel hungry.

That probably means you need food for energy. But you have to give yourself this waiting period because otherwise, your mind might be trying to trick you into just eating something you are craving when you are not genuinely hungry.

There is a mental component to this change in diet, too. The problem at the center of women not being able to change their diet is not being used to the real feeling of being full.

By the "real" feeling of being full, I am referring to how people feel when they have eaten enough—not too much.

These days, people eat so many carbs that their idea of fullness is the uncomfortable feeling they have when they eat too many carbs. But you can't lose weight if you see fullness this way. You will consistently overstuff yourself, believing you are making yourself full when you are actually gorging yourself.

To remind yourself what fullness actually feels like, get used to eating without overstuffing yourself. Get used to not feeling uncomfortable after eating. It can feel strangely comforting to be overstuffed with carbs, but that is not a feeling we can let ourselves get used to. If we do, we will never be happy with the simple feeling of fullness.

As I keep emphasizing, we can't villainize fat anymore. The real problem is eating too many calories, most of which tend to come from carbs, not fats. However, women over 50, in particular, need to be careful not to eat too many fats when they follow Keto.

Keto isn't a valid excuse for simply eating a ton of fat. You still need to show some constraint as you do in every diet.

Understanding how to balance your fat consumption will take an understanding of how fat fits into Keto. With Keto, you want to be what we call fat adapted.

You already know what this means; it is just another way of saying what happens in Ketosis. Being fat-adapted means, you are burning fat for energy with Ketones instead of burning glucose with carbs.

I tell you this term because you should eat a lot of healthy fats until you go through significant Ketosis—until you are fat-adapted. Once that happens, you should start being more careful with how much fat you are consuming.

One of the sources women over 50 will get fat from is drinks. Even the drinks you make at home like coffee with milk can be a lot higher in fat than you think. It should go without saying that the specialty coffee you get topped with whipped cream is high in fat.

Women over 50 know they have their own hurdles to overcome when they chase the goals of weight loss and improved overall health with Keto. But they can do all they can possibly do by following along with the advice in this phase.

Food List

Foods to Eat

The Good Fats

Add Extra-Virgin Olive Oil (EVOO): Olive oil dates back for centuries to a time where oil was used for anointing kings and priests. It's a high-quality oil maintaining low acidity, which makes this oil have a smoke argument as high as 410° Fahrenheit. Which is taller than utmost cooking requests call for, creating olive oil is more stable than other cooking fats. It contains zero carbs for two teaspoons.

Monounsaturated fats, such as the ones in olive oil, are also linked with better blood sugar regulation, including lower fasting glucose and reducing inflammation throughout the body. Olive oil also aids to avoid cardiovascular illness by caring about the integrity of your vascular system and dropping LDL, which is also called your 'bad' cholesterol.

Add Macadamia Oil: One of the benefits of this oil is its high smoke point of 390° Fahrenheit. It carries a mild flavor, which is a super alternative for olive oil in mayonnaise.

Other Monounsaturated & Saturated Fats*: Include* these *items (listed in grams):*

- Organic red palm oil, Avocado, Sesame, Olive, & Flaxseed Oil–Unsalted butter, Chicken fat, Duck fat, & Beef tallow (1 tbsp. – 0 net carbs)
- Ghee–1 tsp. (0)
- Olives (3 jumbo - 5 large/10 small – 1 net carb)
- Unsweetened flaked coconut (3 tbsp. – 2 net carbs)

Dairy & Your Diet

Before beginning the keto way of life, you need to understand dairy and dairy products, which are an essential part of the ketogenic methods. If you're lactose intolerant, maybe the plan isn't for you. The amounts should be monitored to no more than four ounces daily. Choose dairy products that have been cultured and are keto-friendly. The number one choice is unsweetened almond milk. You can also choose from hemp milk and flax milk.

Do you know the difference between butter and ghee? Butter consists of water, milk solids, and butterfat, whereas ghee, an Indian staple, includes pure butterfat. Therefore, if you have lactose sensitivities, ghee is probably your best choice. The ghee also contains medium-chain fatty acids that assist your immune system and digestion.

Calcium

- Broccoli rabe–cooked: 3.5-ounce portion = 120 mg per 100grams
- Greens (spinach, kale, etc.) cooked: 3.5-ounce portion = 135 mg per 100grams
- Sesame seeds: 1-ounce portion = 273 mg per 28grams
- Almond milk (calcium-fortified): 8-ounce portion = 300-450 mg per 225grams
- Almonds: 1-ounce portion = 74 mg per 28grams

Omega 3 Fatty Acids Options

Alpha-linolenic acid (ALA) is the most common omega-3 fatty acid in your diet. The acid content is found in these using one tablespoon portions:

- Chia Seeds: 2.5grams per 14-gram portion
- Ground Flaxseed: 1.6grams per 7-gram portion
- Hemp Seeds: 2grams per 20-gram portion

Iron Options

Be sure you have adequate iron in your diet. Include these food groups:

- Cooked spinach: 3.5-ounce portion = 3.6 mg per 100grams
- Cooked white mushrooms: 3.5-ounce portion = 2.7 mg per 100grams
- Olives: 3.5 oz. portion = 3.3 mg per 100grams
- Sesame seeds: 1-ounce portion = 4.1 mg per 28grams
- Pumpkin seeds: 1-ounce portion = 4.2 mg per 28grams
- Chia seeds: 1-ounce portion = 2.2 mg per 28grams
- Coconut milk: 3.5 oz. portion = 3.3 mg per 100grams
- Canned hearts of palm: 3.5 oz. portion = 3.1 mg per 100grams
- Dark chocolate: 1-ounce portion = 3.3 mg per 28grams

Save Additional Carbohydrates

- *Pasta:* Replace pasta using zucchini. Use a spiralizer and make long ribbons to cover your plate. It is excellent for many dishes served this way. You can also prepare spaghetti squash for regular spaghetti.
- *French Fries:* Change over to zucchini fries or turnip fries.
- *Tortillas:* Get ready to push this one to the side, which weighs in at approximately 98grams for one serving. Instead, enjoy a lettuce leaf at about 1gram per serving.
- *Mashed Potatoes:* There's no need to prepare bowls of regular mashed potatoes; instead, enjoy some mashed cauliflower.

Foods to Avoid

The Limited "Bad" Fats

You need to be aware of unhealthy, processed trans fats and polyunsaturated fats. These facts are acquired through processing and are found in foods, including fast foods, crackers, margarine, and cookies. Avoid canola, soybean, safflower, and cottonseed vegetable oils. If the oil was processed in a factory and prepackaged, you need to be aware of its fat content.

Processed Foods: Don't purchase any items if you see carrageenan on the label. Like so many other people, you shouldn't feel too guilty if you crave all of those processed foods. It happens!

Generally, look for labels with the least amount of ingredients. Usually, the ones that provide the most nutrition are listed in those shorter lists.

Here are just a few of the items you may not realize are loaded with carbs:

Bread, pasta, pizza crusts, or crackers and cookies made with these grains:

- Barley: 44 carbs - 4 protein - 1gram of fat
- Buckwheat: 33 carbs - 6 protein - 1gram of fat
- Wheat: 14 carbs - 3 protein - 1gram of fat
- Corn: 32 carbs - 4 protein - 1gram of fat
- Millet: 41 carbs - 6 protein - 2grams fat
- Oats: 36 carbs - 6 protein - 3grams fat
- Rice: 45 carbs - 5 protein - 2grams fat
- Rye: 15 carbs - 3 protein - 1gram of fat

Watch out for the Sugar Products also:

- Raw Sugar: 12grams of carbs
- High-Fructose Corn Syrup: 14grams of carbs
- Honey: 17grams of carbs
- Maple Syrup: 14grams of carbs
- Cane Sugar: 12grams of carbs

Some of the foods are surprising because they were deemed for years as a healthy and nutritious snacks. I bet you see a few of the culprits that will beckon you onto the wrong path:

- Cereal Bars
- Rice Cakes
- Protein Bars
- Potato Chips
- Flavored Nuts
- Popcorn
- Pretzels
- Crackers

35 Days (5-Weeks) Meal Plan

First Week

Food Plan for the First Week

Day	Breakfast	Lunch	Dinner
1	Sheet Pan Eggs with Veggies and Parmesan	Caprese Zoodles	Slow Roasting Pork Shoulder
2	Kale Avocado Smoothie	Zucchini Sushi	Garlicky Pork Shoulder
3	Almond Butter Protein Smoothie	Asian Chicken Lettuce Wraps	Rosemary Pork Roast
4	Beets and Blueberry Smoothie	California Burger Bowls	Winter Season Pork Dish
5	Almond Butter Muffins	Parmesan Brussels Sprouts Salad	Celebrating Pork Tenderloin
6	Classic Western Omelet	Hot Spicy Chicken	Mustard Pork Tenderloin
7	Sheet Pan Eggs with Ham and Pepper Jack	Broccoli and Turkey Dish	Succulent Pork Tenderloin

Recipes for Breakfast

Sheet Pan Eggs with Veggies and Parmesan

Preparation Time: 5 Minutes

Cooking Time: 15 Minutes

Servings: 2

Ingredients:
- 3 large eggs, whisked
- Salt and pepper
- 1/2 small red pepper, diced
- 1/2 small yellow onion, chopped
- 1/4 cup diced mushrooms
- 1/4 cup diced zucchini
- 1/4 cup freshly grated parmesan cheese

Directions:
1. Preheat the oven to 350°F and grease cooking spray on a rimmed baking sheet.
2. In a cup, whisk the eggs with salt and pepper until sparkling.
3. Remove the peppers, onions, mushrooms, and courgettes until well mixed.
4. Pour the mixture into the baking sheet and scatter over a layer of evenness.
5. Sprinkle with parmesan, and bake until the egg is set for 13 to 16 minutes.
6. Let it cool down slightly, then cut to squares for serving.

Nutrition:
- Calories: 180
- Fat: 10g
- Protein: 14.5g
- Carbohydrates: 5g
- Fiber: 1g
- Net carbs: 4g

Kale Avocado Smoothie

Preparation Time: 5 Minutes

Cooking Time: 0 Minutes

Servings: 2

Ingredients:
- 2 cups fresh chopped kale
- 1 cup chopped avocado
- 1 1/2 cup unsweetened almond milk
- 1/2 cup full-fat yogurt, plain
- 6 to 8 ice cubes
- 2 tablespoons fresh lemon juice
- Liquid stevia extract, to taste

Directions:
1. Combine the kale, avocado, and almond milk in a blender.
2. Pulse the ingredients several times.
3. Add the remaining ingredients and blend them until smooth.
4. Pour into a large glass and enjoy immediately.

Nutrition:
- Calories: 250
- Fat: 19g
- Protein: 6g
- Carbs: 17.5g
- Fiber: 6.5g
- Net carbs: 11g

Almond Butter Protein Smoothie	Beets and Blueberry Smoothie
Preparation Time: 5 Minutes	**Preparation Time:** 5 Minutes
Cooking Time: 0 Minutes	**Cooking Time:** 0 Minutes
Servings: 2	**Servings:** 2

Almond Butter Protein Smoothie

Ingredients:

- 2 cups unsweetened almond milk
- 1 cup full-fat yogurt, plain
- 1/2 cup vanilla egg white protein powder
- 2 tablespoons almond butter
- Pinch ground cinnamon
- Liquid stevia extract, to taste

Directions:

1. In a blender, add the almond milk and yogurt.
2. Pulse several times over the ingredients.
3. Stir in the remaining ingredients and blend until smooth.
4. Pour into a big glass, and instantly enjoy it.

Nutrition:

- Calories: 315
- Fat: 16.5g
- Protein: 31.5g
- Carbohydrates: 12g
- Sugar: 2,5g
- Net carb: 9,5g

Beets and Blueberry Smoothie

Ingredients:

- 2 cups unsweetened coconut milk
- 1/2 cup heavy cream
- 1/2 cup frozen blueberries
- 2 small beets, peeled and chopped
- 2 teaspoons chia seeds
- Liquid stevia extract, to taste

Directions:

1. In a blender, add the blueberries, beets, and coconut milk.
2. Pulse several times over the ingredients.
3. Stir in the remaining ingredients and blend until smooth.
4. Pour into a big glass, and instantly enjoy it.

Nutrition:

- Calories: 215
- Fat: 17g
- Protein: 2.5g
- Carbohydrates: 15g
- Fiber: 5g
- Net carbs: 10g

Almond Butter Muffins

Preparation Time: 10 Minutes

Cooking Time: 25 Minutes

Servings: 2

Ingredients:
- 1 cup almond flour
- 1/2 cup powdered erythritol
- 1 teaspoons baking powder
- ¼ teaspoon salt
- ¾ cup almond butter, warmed
- ¾ cup unsweetened almond milk
- 2 eggs

Directions:
1. Preheat the oven to 350°F, and line a paper liner muffin pan.
2. In a mixing bowl, whisk the almond flour and the erythritol, baking powder, and salt.
3. Whisk the almond milk, almond butter, and eggs together in a separate bowl.
4. Drop the wet ingredients into the dry until just mixed together.
5. Spoon the batter into the prepared pan and bake for 22 to 25 minutes until clean comes out the knife inserted in the middle.
6. Cook the muffins in the pan for 5 minutes. Then, switch onto a cooling rack with wire.

Nutrition:
- Calories: 135
- Fat: 11g
- Protein: 6g
- Carbohydrates: 4g
- Fiber: 2g
- Net carbs: 2g

Classic Western Omelet

Preparation Time: 5 Minutes

Cooking Time: 10 Minutes

Servings: 2

Ingredients:
- 1 teaspoon coconut oil
- 3 large eggs, whisked
- 1 tablespoon heavy cream
- Salt and pepper
- ¼ cup diced green pepper
- ¼ cup diced yellow onion
- ¼ cup diced ham

Directions:
1. In a small bowl, whisk the eggs, heavy cream, salt, and pepper.
2. Heat up 1 teaspoon of coconut oil over medium heat in a small skillet.
3. Add the peppers and onions, then sauté the ham for 3 to 4 minutes.
4. Spoon the mixture in a cup, and heat the skillet with the remaining oil.
5. Pour in the whisked eggs and cook until the egg's bottom begins to set.
6. Tilt the pan and cook until almost set to spread the egg.
7. Spoon the ham and veggie mixture over half of the omelet and turn over.
8. Let cook the omelet until the eggs are set and then serve hot.

Nutrition:
- Calories: 415
- Fat: 32,5g
- Protein: 25g
- Carbs: 6,5g
- Sugar: 1,5g
- Carbs net: 5g

Sheet Pan Eggs with Ham and Pepper Jack

Preparation Time: 5 Minutes

Cooking Time: 15 Minutes

Servings: 2

Ingredients:
- 4 large eggs, whisked
- Salt and pepper
- 1/2 cup diced ham
- 1/2 cup shredded pepper jack cheese

Directions:
1. Preheat the oven to 350°F and grease a rimmed baking sheet with cooking spray.
2. Whisk the eggs in a mixing bowl then add salt and pepper until frothy.
3. Stir in the ham and cheese and mix until well combined.
4. Pour the mixture into baking sheets and spread it into an even layer.
5. Bake for 12 to 15 mins until the egg is set.
6. Let cool slightly then cut it into squares to serve.

Nutrition:
- Calories: 235
- Fat: 15g
- Protein: 21g
- Carbs: 2.5g
- Fiber: 0.5g
- Net carbs: 2g

Recipes for Lunch

Caprese Zoodles

Preparation Time: 15 Minutes

Cooking Time: 0 Minutes

Servings: 2

Ingredients:
- 2 zucchinis
- 1 tbsp. extra-virgin olive oil
- Kosher salt
- Ground black pepper
- 1 c. cherry tomatoes halved
- 1/2 c. mozzarella balls
- 1/8 c. basil leaves
- 1 tbsp. balsamic vinegar

Directions:
1. Creating zoodles out of zucchini using a spiralizer.
2. Mix the zoodles, olive oil, salt, and pepper. Marinate for 15 minutes.
3. Put the tomatoes, mozzarella, and basil and toss.
4. Drizzle, and drink with balsamic vinegar.

Nutrition:
- Calories: 417
- Carbohydrates: 11g
- Fat: 24g
- Protein: 36g

Zucchini Sushi

Preparation Time: 20 Minutes

Cooking Time: 0 Minutes

Servings: 2

Ingredients:
- 2 zucchinis
- 4 oz. cream cheese
- 1 tsp. Sriracha hot sauce
- 1 tsp. lime juice
- 1 c. lump crab meat
- 1/2 carrot
- 1/2 avocado
- 1/2 cucumber
- 1 tsp. toasted sesame seeds

Directions:
1. Slice each zucchini into thin flat strips. Put aside.
2. Combine cream cheese, sriracha, and lime juice in a medium-sized cup.
3. Place two slices of zucchini horizontally flat on a cutting board.
4. Place a lean layer of cream cheese over it, then top the left with a slice of lobster, carrot, avocado, and cucumber.
5. Roll up zucchini. Serve with sesame seeds.

Nutrition:
- Calories: 450
- Carbohydrates: 23g
- Fat: 25g
- Protein: 35g

Asian Chicken Lettuce Wraps

Preparation Time: 15 Minutes

Cooking Time: 15 Minutes

Servings: 2

Ingredients:

- 1/2 tbsp. hoisin sauce
- 1 tbsp. low-sodium soy sauce
- 1 tbsp. rice wine vinegar
- 1/2 tbsp. Sriracha
- 1/2 tsp. sesame oil
- 1/2 tbsp. extra-virgin olive oil
- 1/2 onion
- 1 garlic clove
- 1/2 tbsp. grated ginger
- 1/2 lb. ground chicken
- 1/4 c. water chestnuts
- 1 green onion
- Kosher salt
- Ground black pepper
- Large leafy lettuce
- Cooked white rice

Directions:

1. To make the sauce, mix the hoisin sauce, soy sauce, rice wine vinegar, sriracha, and sesame oil in a small bowl.
2. Mix the olive oil in a large pan.
3. Put onions and cook within 5 minutes, then stir in garlic and ginger and cook for 1 minute.
4. Put ground chicken and cook.
5. Put in the sauce and cook within 1 to 2 minutes.
6. Turn off the heat and put in the green onions and chestnuts. Season with pepper and salt.
7. Add spoon rice of chicken mixture in the center of a lettuce leaf. Serve.

Nutrition:

- Calories: 315
- Carbohydrates: 5g
- Fat: 12g
- Protein: 34g

California Burger Bowls

Preparation Time: 15 Minutes
Cooking Time: 20 Minutes
Servings: 2

Ingredients:
For the dressing:

- 1/4 c. extra-virgin olive oil
- 1/6 c. balsamic vinegar
- 1 1/2 tbsp. Dijon mustard
- 1 tsp. honey
- 1/2 clove garlic
- Kosher salt
- Ground black pepper

For the burger:

- 1/2 lb. grass-fed organic ground beef
- 1/2 tsp. Worcestershire sauce
- 1/4 tsp. chili powder
- 1/4 tsp. onion powder
- Kosher salt
- Ground black pepper
- 1/2 package butterhead lettuce
- 1/2 medium red onion
- 1/2 avocado
- 1 tomato

Directions:

1. To make the dressing, mix the dressing items in a medium bowl.
2. To make burgers, combine beef and Worcestershire sauce, chili powder, and onion powder in another large bowl. Put pepper and salt, mix.
3. Form into four patties.
4. Grill the onions within 3 minutes each. Remove and detach burgers from the grill pan. Cook within 4 minutes per side.
5. To plate, put lettuce in a large bowl with 1/2 the dressing. Finish with a patty burger, grilled onions, 1/4 slices of avocado, and tomatoes. Serve.

Nutrition:

- Calories: 407
- Carbohydrates: 33g
- Fat: 19g
- Protein: 26g

Parmesan Brussels Sprouts Salad

Preparation Time: 15 Minutes

Cooking Time: 25 Minutes

Servings: 2

Ingredients:
- 2 tbsp. extra-virgin olive oil
- 2 tbsp. lemon juice
- 1/4 c. parsley
- Kosher salt
- Ground black pepper
- 1/2 lb. Brussels sprouts
- 1/4 c. toasted almonds
- 1/4 c. pomegranate seeds
- Shaved Parmesan

Directions:
1. Mix olive oil, lemon juice, parsley, two teaspoons of salt, and one teaspoon of pepper.
2. Add the Brussels sprouts in and toss.
3. Let sit before serving within 20 minutes and up to 4 hours.
4. Fold in almonds and pomegranate seeds and garnish with a rasped parmesan. Serve.

Nutrition:
- Calories: 130
- Carbohydrates: 8g
- Fat: 9g
- Protein: 4g

Hot Spicy Chicken

Preparation Time: 5 Minutes

Cooking Time: 25 Minutes

Servings: 2

Ingredients:
- ¼ tbsp fennel seeds, ground
- ¼ tsp smoked paprika
- ½ tsp hot paprika
- ½ tsp minced garlic
- 2 chicken thighs, boneless

Directions:
1. Preheat the oven to 325°F.
2. To prepare the spice mix, add all the ingredients in a small bowl except for chicken. Stir until well mixed.
3. Brush the mixture on all sides of the chicken, rub it well into the meat, then place the chicken onto a baking sheet.
4. Roast for 15 to 25 minutes until thoroughly cooked, basting every 10 minutes with the drippings.

Nutrition:
- Calories: 102.3
- Fats: 8g
- Protein: 7.2g
- Net Carb: 0.3g
- Fiber: 0.3g

Broccoli and Turkey Dish

Preparation Time: 5 Minutes

Cooking Time: 15 Minutes

Servings: 2

Ingredients:
- ¼ tsp red pepper flakes
- 1 tbsp olive oil
- 1 tsp soy sauce
- 4 oz broccoli florets
- 4 oz cauliflower florets, riced
- 4 oz ground turkey

Directions:
1. Bring out a skillet pan, place it over medium heat.
2. Add olive oil and when hot, add beef. Crumble it and cook for 8 minutes until no longer pink.
3. Then add broccoli florets and riced cauliflower. Stir well, drizzle with soy sauce and sesame oil, season with salt, black pepper, and red pepper flakes.
4. Continue cooking for 5 minutes until vegetables have been thoroughly cooked.

Nutrition:
- Calories: 120.3
- Fats: 8.3g
- Protein: 8.4g
- Net Carb: 2g
- Fiber: 1g

Recipes for Dinner

Slow Roasting Pork Shoulder

Preparation Time: 15 Minutes

Cooking Time: 7 Hours

Servings: 2

Ingredients:
- 1/2 lb. pork shoulder
- 1garlic clove, minced
- 1/4 C. fresh lemon juice
- 1/2 tbsp. olive oil
- 1/2 tbsp. low-sodium soy sauce
- 1/4 C. homemade chicken broth

Directions:
1. In a nonreactive baking dish, arrange the pork shoulder, fat side up. With the tip of the knife, score the fat in a crosshatch pattern.
2. In a bowl, add the garlic, lemon juice, soy sauce, and oil and mix well. Place the marinade over pork and coat well.
3. Refrigerate for about 4-6 hours, flipping occasionally. Preheat the oven to 315°F. Lightly grease a large roasting pan.
4. With paper towels, wipe marinade off the pork shoulder. Arrange the pork shoulder into a prepared roasting pan, fat side up.
5. Roast for about 3 hours. Remove from the oven and pour the broth over the pork shoulder.
6. Roast for about 3-4 hours, basting with pan juices, after every 1 hour. Remove from the oven and place the pork shoulder onto a cutting board for about 30 minutes. Slice and serve.

Nutrition:
- Calories: 537
- Carbs: 1.5g
- Protein: 40.2g
- Fat: 40.1g
- Sugar: 0.5g
- Sodium: 261mg
- Fiber: 0.1g

Garlicky Pork Shoulder

Preparation Time: 15 Minutes

Cooking Time: 6 Hours

Servings: 2

Ingredients:
- 2garlic cloves, peeled and crushed
- 1/8 C. fresh rosemary, minced
- 1/2 tbsp. fresh lemon juice
- 1/2 tbsp. balsamic vinegar
- 1 (1/2-lb.) pork shoulder

Directions:
1. Put all the fixings except pork shoulder in a bowl and mix well. Put the pork shoulder in your roasting pan and generously coat with the marinade.
2. With a large plastic wrap, cover the roasting pan and refrigerate to marinate for at least 1-2 hours.
3. Remove the roasting pan from the refrigerator. Remove the plastic wrap from the roasting pan and keep it at room temperature for 1 hour.
4. Preheat the oven to 275°F. Place the roasting pan into the oven and roast for about 6 hours.
5. Remove from the oven and place pork shoulder onto a cutting board for about 30 minutes. Slice and serve.

Nutrition:
- Calories: 502
- Carbs: 2g
- Protein: 42.5g
- Fat: 39.1g
- Sugar: 0.1g
- Sodium: 125mg
- Fiber: 0.7g

Rosemary Pork Roast

Preparation Time: 15 Minutes
Cooking Time: 60 Minutes
Servings: 2

Ingredients:
- 1/2 tbsp. dried rosemary, crushed
- 1garlic clove, minced
- Salt
- Ground black pepper
- 1/2 lb. boneless pork loin roast
- 1 tsp olive oil
- 1/8 C. homemade chicken broth

Directions:
1. Preheat the oven to 350ºF, then grease a roasting pan.
2. Put rosemary, garlic, salt, and black pepper in a small bowl and crush it to form a paste.
3. Prick the pork loin at all places, then press the half of rosemary batter into the cuts.
4. Put oil in the bowl with the rest of the rosemary mixture to mix and massage the pork with it.
5. Roast within 1 hour, flipping and coating with the pan juices occasionally.
6. Remove, then transfer the pork to a serving platter. Place the roasting pan over medium heat.
7. Add the broth and cook for about 3-5 minutes, stirring to lose the brown bits. Pour sauce over pork and serve.

Nutrition:
- Calories: 294
- Carbs: 0.9g
- Protein: 40g
- Fat: 13.9g
- Sugar: 0.1g
- Sodium: 156mg
- Fiber: 0.3g

Winter Season Pork Dish

Preparation Time: 15 Minutes
Cooking Time: 2 Hours
Servings: 2

Ingredients:
- 6 oz. sauerkraut
- 1/2 lb. pork roast
- Salt
- Ground black pepper
- 1/8 C. unsalted butter
- 1/2 yellow onion, sliced thinly
- 3 oz. precooked kielbasa, cut into ½-inch rounds

Directions:
1. Preheat the oven to 325ºF.
2. Drain the sauerkraut, reserving about 1 C. of liquid. Rub the pork roast with salt plus black pepper.
3. In a heavy-bottomed skillet, melt the butter over high heat and sear the pork for about 5-6 minutes per side.
4. With a slotted spoon, transfer the pork onto a plate. At the bottom of a casserole, place half of sauerkraut and onion slices.
5. Place the seared pork roast and kielbasa pieces on top. Top with the remaining sauerkraut and onion slices.
6. Pour the reserved sauerkraut liquid into the casserole dish. Cover the casserole dish tightly and bake for about 2 hours.
7. Remove from the oven, and with tongs, transfer the pork roast onto a cutting board for at least 15 minutes. With a sharp knife, cut the pork roast into desired size slices.
8. Divide the pork slices onto serving plates and serve alongside the sauerkraut mixture.

Nutrition:
- Calories: 417
- Carbs: 6.3g
- Protein: 39g
- Fat: 25g
- Sugar: 2g
- Sodium: 1200mg
- Fiber: 3g

Celebrating Pork Tenderloin

Preparation Time: 15 Minutes
Cooking Time: 40 Minutes
Servings: 2
Ingredients:
For Pork Tenderloin:

- 1 garlic clove, minced
- 1/2 tsp. dried rosemary, crushed
- 1/8 tsp. cayenne pepper
- Salt
- Ground black pepper
- 1/2 lb. pork tenderloin

For Blueberry Sauce:

- 1/2 tbsp. olive oil
- 1/2 yellow onion, chopped
- 1/4 tsp. Erythritol
- 1/8 C. organic apple cider vinegar
- 1/2 C. fresh blueberries
- 1/8 tsp. dried thyme, crushed
- Salt
- Ground black pepper, to taste

Directions:

1. Preheat the oven to 400ºF. Grease a roasting pan.
2. For the pork: in a bowl, mix all the ingredients except pork. Rub the pork with garlic mixture evenly.
3. Place the pork into the prepared roasting pan. Roast for about 25 minutes or until desired doneness.
4. Meanwhile, in a pan, for sauce, heat the oil over medium-high heat and sauté the onion for about 4-5 minutes. Stir in the remaining ingredients and cook for about 7-8 minutes or until desired thickness, stirring frequently.
5. Remove and place the pork tenderloin onto a cutting board for about 10-15 minutes. With a sharp knife, cut the pork tenderloin into desired size slices and serve with the topping of blueberry sauce.

Nutrition:

- Calories: 276
- Sugar: 5g
- Carbs: 9g
- Sodium: 116mg
- Protein: 40g
- Fiber: 2g
- Fat: 8g

Mustard Pork Tenderloin

Preparation Time: 15 Minutes
Cooking Time: 30 Minutes

Servings: 2

Ingredients:

- 1/2 tsp. fresh rosemary, minced
- 1garlic clove, minced
- 1/2 tbsp. fresh lemon juice
- 1/2 tbsp. olive oil
- 1/2 tsp. Dijon mustard
- 1/2 tsp. powdered Swerve
- Salt
- Ground black pepper
- 1/2 lb. pork tenderloin
- 1/8 C. blue cheese, crumbled

Directions:

1. Preheat oven to 400ºF. Grease a large rimmed baking sheet.
2. Put all the fixings except the pork tenderloin and cheese in a large bowl and beat until well combined.
3. Put the pork tenderloin, then coat with the mixture generously. Arrange the pork tenderloin onto the prepared baking sheet.
4. Bake for about 20-22 minutes. Remove from the oven and place the pork tenderloin onto a cutting board for about 5 minutes.
5. With a sharp knife, cut the pork tenderloin into ¾-inch thick slices and serve with cheese topping.

Nutrition:

- Calories: 227
- Carbs: 2g
- Protein: 37g
- Fat: 10g
- Sugar: 0.5g
- Sodium: 236mg
- Fiber: 0.1g

Succulent Pork Tenderloin

Preparation Time: 20 Minutes

Cooking Time: 60 Minutes

Servings: 2

Ingredients:
- 1/2 lb. pork tenderloin
- 1/2 tbsp. unsalted butter
- 1 tsp. garlic, minced
- 1 oz. fresh spinach
- 2 oz. cream cheese softened
- 1/2 tsp. liquid smoke
- Salt
- Ground black pepper

Directions:
1. Preheat the oven to 350°F. Line the casserole dish with a piece of foil.
2. Arrange the pork tenderloin between 2 plastic wraps and with a meat tenderizer, pound until flat. Carefully cut the edges of the tenderloin to shape into a rectangle.
3. Dissolve the butter over medium heat in a large skillet and sauté the garlic for about 1 minute.
4. Add the spinach, cream cheese, liquid smoke, salt, and black pepper, and cook for about 3-4 minutes.
5. Remove and set aside to cool slightly. Place the spinach mixture onto pork tenderloin about ½-inch from the edges.
6. Carefully roll tenderloin into a log and secure with toothpicks. Arrange the tenderloin into the prepared casserole dish, seam-side down.
7. Bake for about 1¼ hours. Remove from the oven and let it cool slightly before cutting. Cut the tenderloin into desired sized slices and serve.

Nutrition:
- Calories: 315
- Protein: 43g
- Sugar: 0.5g
- Fiber: 0.1g
- Carbs: 3g
- Fat: 23g
- Sodium: 261mg

Second Week

Food Plan for the Second Week

Day	Breakfast	Lunch	Dinner
1	Detoxifying Green Smoothie	Easy Mayo Salmon	Simple Ever Rib Roast
2	Tomato Mozzarella Egg Muffins	Keto Buffalo Chicken Empanadas	Family Dinner Tenderloin
3	Crispy Chai Waffles	Pepperoni and Cheddar Stromboli	Tex-Mex Casserole
4	Nutty Pumpkin Smoothie	Zesty Avocado and Lettuce Salad	Keto Chicken and Roasted Veggies
5	Broccoli, Kale, Egg Scramble	Veggie, Bacon, and Egg Dish	Salmon Pie
6	Creamy Chocolate Protein Smoothie	Keto Teriyaki Chicken	Keto Falafel
7	Three Cheese Egg Muffins	Lime Chicken with Coleslaw	Ham Croquettes

Recipes for Breakfast

Detoxifying Green Smoothie

Preparation Time: 5 Minutes

Cooking Time: 0 Minutes

Servings: 2

Ingredients:
- 2 cups fresh chopped kale
- 1 cup fresh baby spinach
- 1/2 cup sliced celery
- 1/2 cup water
- 6 to 8 ice cubes
- 4 tablespoons fresh lemon juice
- 2 tablespoons fresh lime juice
- 2 tablespoons coconut oil
- Liquid stevia extract, to taste

Directions:
1. In a blender, add the broccoli, spinach, and celery.
2. Pulse several times over the ingredients.
3. Stir in the remaining ingredients and blend until smooth.
4. Pour into a big glass, and instantly enjoy it.

Nutrition:
- Calories: 160
- Fat: 14g
- Protein: 2.5g
- Carbs: 8g

Nutty Pumpkin Smoothie

Preparation Time: 5 Minutes

Cooking Time: 0 Minutes

Servings: 2

Ingredients:
- 2 cups unsweetened cashew milk
- 1 cup pumpkin puree
- 1/2 cup heavy cream
- 2 tablespoons raw almonds
- 1/2 tcaspoon pumpkin pie spice
- Liquid stevia extract, to taste

Directions:
1. Combine all of the ingredients in a blender.
2. Pulse the ingredients several times, then blend until smooth.
3. Pour into a large glass and enjoy immediately.

Nutrition:
- Calories: 205
- Fat: 16.5g
- Protein: 3g
- Carbs: 13g
- Fiber: 4.5g
- Net carbs: 8.5g

Tomato Mozzarella Egg Muffins

Preparation Time: 5 Minutes

Cooking Time: 25 Minutes

Servings: 2

Ingredients:
- 1/2 tablespoon butter
- 1 medium tomato, finely diced
- ½ cup diced yellow onion
- 2 large eggs, whisked
- 1/4 cup canned coconut milk
- ¼ cup sliced green onion
- Salt and pepper
- 1/2 cup shredded mozzarella cheese

Directions:
1. Preheat the oven to 350°F and grease the cooking spray into a muffin pan.
2. Melt the butter over moderate heat in a medium skillet.
3. Add the tomato and onions, then cook until softened for 3 to 4 minutes.
4. Divide the mix between cups of muffins.
5. Whisk the bacon, coconut milk, green onions, salt, and pepper together, and then spoon into the muffin cups.
6. Sprinkle with cheese until the egg is set, then bake for 15 to 25 minutes.

Nutrition:
- Calories: 135
- Fat: 10.5g
- Protein: 9g
- Carbs: 2g
- Fiber: 0.5g
- Net carbs: 1.5g

Crispy Chai Waffles

Preparation Time: 10 Minutes
Cooking Time: 20 Minutes
Servings: 2
Ingredients:
- 2 large eggs, separated into whites and yolks
- 2 tablespoons coconut flour
- 2 tablespoons powdered erythritol
- 3/4 teaspoon baking powder
- 1/2 teaspoon vanilla extract
- 1/4 teaspoon ground cinnamon
- ¼ teaspoon ground ginger
- Pinch ground cloves
- Pinch ground cardamom
- 1 tablespoon coconut oil, melted
- 1 tablespoon unsweetened almond milk

Directions:
1. Divide the eggs into two separate mixing bowls.
2. Whip the whites of the eggs until stiff peaks develop and then set aside.
3. Whisk the egg yolks into the other bowl with the coconut flour, erythritol, baking powder, cocoa, cinnamon, cardamom, and cloves.
4. Pour the melted coconut oil and the almond milk into the second bowl and whisk.
5. Fold softly in the whites of the egg until you have just combined.
6. Preheat waffle iron with cooking spray and grease.
7. Spoon into the iron for about 1/2 cup of batter.
8. Cook the waffle according to directions from the maker.
9. Move the waffle to a plate and repeat with the batter left over.

Nutrition:
- Calories: 215
- Fat: 17g
- Protein: 8g
- Carbohydrates: 8g
- Fiber: 4g
- Net carbs: 4g

Broccoli, Kale, Egg Scramble

Preparation Time: 5 Minutes

Cooking Time: 10 Minutes

Servings: 2

Ingredients:
- 2 large eggs, whisked
- 1 tablespoon heavy cream
- Salt and pepper
- 1 teaspoon coconut oil
- 1 cup fresh chopped kale
- ¼ cup frozen broccoli florets, thawed
- 2 tablespoons grated parmesan cheese

Directions:
1. In a mug, whisk the eggs along with the heavy cream, salt, and pepper.
2. Heat 1 teaspoon coconut oil over medium heat in a medium-size skillet.
3. Stir in the kale and broccoli, then cook about 1 to 2 minutes until the kale is wilted.
4. Pour in the eggs and cook until just set, stirring occasionally.
5. Stir in the cheese with parmesan and serve hot.

Nutrition:
- Calories: 315
- Fat: 23g
- Protein: 19.5g
- Carbs: 10g
- Fiber: 1.5g
- Net carbs: 8.5g

Creamy Chocolate Protein Smoothie

Preparation Time: 5 Minutes

Cooking Time: 0 Minutes

Servings: 2

Ingredients:
- 2 cups unsweetened almond milk
- 1 cup full-fat yogurt, plain
- 1/2 cup chocolate egg white protein powder
- 2 tablespoons coconut oil
- 2 tablespoons unsweetened cocoa powder
- Liquid stevia extract, to taste

Directions:
1. In a blender, add the almond milk, yogurt, and protein powder.
2. Pulse several times on the ingredients then add the rest and blend until smooth.
3. Pour into a big glass, and instantly enjoy it.

Nutrition:
- Calories: 345
- Fat: 22g
- Protein: 29g
- Carbohydrates: 12g
- Fiber: 3g
- Net carbs: 9g

Three Cheese Egg Muffins

Preparation Time: 5 Minutes

Cooking Time: 20 Minutes

Servings: 2

Ingredients:
- 1 tablespoon butter
- ½ cup diced yellow onion
- 3 large eggs, whisked
- 1/2 cup canned coconut milk
- 1/2 cup sliced green onion
- Salt and pepper
- ½ cup shredded cheddar cheese
- ½ cup shredded Swiss cheese
- ¼ cup grated parmesan cheese

Directions:
1. Preheat the oven to 350°F and grease the cooking spray into a muffin pan.
2. Melt the butter over moderate heat in a medium skillet.
3. Add the onions then cook until softened for 3 to 4 minutes.
4. Divide the mix between cups of muffins.
5. Whisk the bacon, coconut milk, green onions, salt, and pepper together, and then spoon into the muffin cups.
6. In a cup, mix the three kinds of cheese, and scatter over the egg muffins.
7. Bake till the egg is set, for 20 to 25 minutes.

Nutrition:
- Calories: 150
- Fat: 11.5g
- Protein: 10g
- Carbs: 2g
- Fiber: 0.5g
- Net carbs: 1.5g

Recipes for Lunch

Easy Mayo Salmon

Preparation Time: 5 Minutes

Cooking Time: 10 Minutes

Servings: 2

Ingredients:
- 2 salmon fillets
- 4 tbsp mayonnaise

Directions:
1. Turn on the panini press, spray it with oil, and let it preheat.
2. Spread 1 tbsp. of mayonnaise on each side of the salmon, place them on Panini press pan, shut with a lid, and cook for 7 to 10 minutes until the salmon has cooked to the desired level.

Nutrition:
- Calories: 132.7
- Fats: 11. 1g
- Protein: 8g
- Net Carb: 0.3g

Keto Buffalo Chicken Empanadas

Preparation Time: 20 Minutes
Cooking Time: 30 Minutes
Servings: 2

Ingredients:
- For the empanada dough
- 3/4 cup mozzarella cheese
- 1 oz cream cheese
- 1 whisked egg
- 1 cup almond flour
- For the buffalo chicken filling
- 1 cup shredded chicken
- 1 tablespoon butter
- 1/4 cup Hot Sauce

Directions:
1. Warm up the oven to 425°F.
2. Microwave the cheese & cream cheese within one minute.
3. Stir the flour and egg into the dish.
4. In another bowl, combine the chicken with sauce and set aside.
5. Cover a flat surface with plastic wrap and sprinkle with almond flour.
6. Grease a rolling pin, press the dough flat.
7. Make the circle shapes out of this dough with a lid.
8. Portion out spoonful of filling into these dough circles.
9. Fold the other half over to close up into half-moon shapes.
10. Bake within 9 minutes. Serve.

Nutrition:
- Calories: 1217kcal
- Net carbohydrates: 20g
- Fiber: 0g
- Fat: 96g
- Protein: 74g

Pepperoni and Cheddar Stromboli

Preparation Time: 15 Minutes

Cooking Time: 20 Minutes

Servings: 2

Ingredients:
- 1.25 cups mozzarella cheese
- 0.25 cup almond flour
- 3 tablespoons coconut flour
- 1 teaspoon Italian seasoning
- 1 egg
- 6 oz deli ham
- 2 oz pepperoni
- 4 oz cheddar cheese
- 1 tbsp butter
- 6 cups salad greens

Directions:
1. Warm up the oven to 400°F.
2. Melt the mozzarella.
3. Mix flours & Italian seasoning in a separate bowl.
4. Dump in the melty cheese and mix with pepper and salt.
5. Stir in the egg and process the dough.
6. Pour it onto that prepared baking tray.
7. Roll out the dough. Cut slits that mark out 4 equal rectangles.
8. Put the ham and cheese, then brush with butter and close up.
9. Bake within 17 minutes. Slice and serve.

Nutrition:
- Net carbohydrates: 20g
- Fiber: 0g
- Fat: 13g
- Protein: 11g
- Calories: 240kcal

Zesty Avocado and Lettuce Salad

Preparation Time: 5 Minutes

Cooking Time: 0 Minutes

Servings: 2

Ingredients:
- ½ of a lime, juiced
- 1 avocado, pitted, sliced
- 2 tbsp olive oil
- 4 oz chopped lettuce
- 4 tbsp chopped chives

Directions:
1. In a small bowl, add oil, lime juice, salt, and black pepper, stir until mixed, and then slowly mix oil until the dressing is combined.
2. Bring out a large bowl, add avocado, lettuce, and chives, and then toss gently.
3. Drizzle with dressing, toss until well coated. Serve.

Nutrition:
- Calories: 125.7
- Fats: 1 1g
- Protein: 1.3g
- Net Carb: 1.7g
- Fiber: 3.7g

Veggie, Bacon, and Egg Dish	Keto Teriyaki Chicken
Preparation Time: 5 Minutes	**Preparation Time:** 5 Minutes
Cooking Time: 5 Minutes	**Cooking Time:** 18 Minutes
Servings: 2	**Servings:** 2

Veggie, Bacon, and Egg Dish

Ingredients:

- ¼ cup mayonnaise
- 2 eggs, boiled, sliced
- 4 oz spinach
- 4 slices of bacon, chopped

Directions:

1. Heat a skillet pan over medium heat, add bacon, and cook for 5 minutes until browned.
2. In a salad bowl, add spinach, top with bacon and eggs, and drizzle with mayonnaise.
3. Toss until well mixed and then serve.

Nutrition:

- Calories: 181.5
- Fats: 16.7g
- Protein: 7.3g
- Net Carb: 0.2g
- Fiber: 0.3g

Keto Teriyaki Chicken

Ingredients:

- 1 tbsp olive oil
- 1 tbsp swerve sweetener
- 2 chicken thighs, boneless
- 2 tbsp soy sauce

Directions:

1. Heat a skillet pan over medium heat.
2. Add oil and when hot, add chicken thighs. Cook for 5 minutes per side until seared.
3. Then sprinkle sugar over chicken thighs, drizzle with soy sauce, and bring the sauce to boil.
4. Switch heat to medium-low level, continue cooking for 3 minutes until chicken is evenly glazed, and then transfer to a plate.
5. Serve chicken with cauliflower rice.

Nutrition:

- Calories: 150
- Fats: 9g
- Protein: 17.3g
- Net Carb: 0g
- Fiber: 0g

Lime Chicken with Coleslaw

Preparation Time: 35 Minutes

Cooking Time: 8 Minutes

Servings: 2

Ingredients:
- ¼ tsp minced garlic
- ½ of a lime, juiced, zested
- ¾ tbsp apple cider vinegar
- 1 chicken thigh, boneless
- 2 oz coleslaw

Directions:
1. Prepare the marinade in a medium bowl. Add vinegar, oil, garlic, paprika, salt, lime juice, and zest. Stir until well mixed.
2. Cut chicken thighs into bite-size pieces, toss until well mixed, and marinate it in the refrigerator for 30 minutes.
3. Heat a skillet pan over medium-high heat, add butter and marinated chicken pieces. Cook for 8 minutes until golden brown and thoroughly cooked.
4. Serve chicken with coleslaw.

Nutrition:
- Calories: 157.3
- Fats: 12.8g
- Protein: 9g
- Net Carb: 1g

Recipes for Dinner

Simple Ever Rib Roast

Preparation Time: 15 Minutes

Cooking Time: 60 Minutes

Servings: 2

Ingredients:
- 2garlic cloves, minced
- 1 tsp. dried thyme, crushed
- 1 tbsp. olive oil
- Salt
- Ground black pepper
- 1 (1/2-lb.) grass-fed prime rib roast

Directions:
1. Mix all the ingredients except rib roast in a bowl. In a large roasting pan, place the rib roast, fatty side up.
2. Coat the rib roast with garlic mixture evenly. Set aside to marinate at room temperature for at least 1 hour.
3. Preheat the oven to 500ºF. Roast for about 20 minutes. Now, lower to 325ºF. Roast for 65-75 minutes.
4. Remove and place the roast onto a cutting board for about 10-15 minutes before slicing. With a sharp knife, cut the rib roast in desired sized slices and serve.

Nutrition:
- Calories: 500
- Carbs: 1g
- Protein: 60g
- Fat: 26g
- Sugar: 0.5g
- Sodium: 200mg
- Fiber: 0.1g

Family Dinner Tenderloin

Preparation Time: 15 Minutes
Cooking Time: 30 Minutes
Servings: 2

Ingredients:
- 1garlic clove, minced
- 1/4 C. fresh parsley, chopped
- 1/4 C. fresh oregano, chopped
- 1 tbsp. fresh thyme, chopped
- 1 tbsp. fresh rosemary, chopped
- 1 tsp. fresh lemon zest, grated
- 1 tbsp. olive oil
- 1 tbsp. fresh lemon juice
- 1/4 tsp. red pepper flakes
- Salt
- Ground black pepper
- 1/2 lb. grass-fed beef tenderloin, silver skin removed

Directions:
1. Put all the ingredients except the beef tenderloin in a large bowl and mix well.
2. Add the beef tenderloin and coat with the herb mixture generously. Refrigerate to marinate for about 30-45 minutes.
3. Preheat the oven to 425ºF. Remove the beef tenderloin from the bowl and arrange it onto a baking sheet.
4. Bake for about 30 minutes. Remove and place the beef tenderloin onto a cutting board for about 15-20 minutes before slicing.
5. With a sharp knife, cut the beef tenderloin into desired sized slices and serve.

Nutrition:
- Calories: 420
- Carbs: 5.2g
- Protein: 40g
- Fat: 27g
- Sugar: 0.5g
- Sodium: 121mg
- Fiber: 3g

Tex-Mex Casserole

Preparation Time: 15 Minutes
Cooking Time: 25 Minutes
Servings: 2

Ingredients:
- 1 pound of beef (ground)
- 1 ounce of butter
- 2 tbsps. of Tex-Mex seasoning
- 3 ounces of tomatoes (crushed)
- 2 ounces of pickled jalapenos
- 3 ounces of cheese (shredded)
- For serving:
- 1/2 cup of sour cream
- 1/2 scallion (chopped)
- 2 ounces of leafy greens
- 1/2 cup of guacamole

Directions:
1. Preheat your oven at two hundred degrees Celsius.
2. Heat butter in an iron skillet. Add the ground beef—Fry for five minutes. Add the crushed tomatoes along with the seasoning, then simmer for five minutes.
3. Pour the beef mixture into a large baking dish. Add cheese and jalapenos—Bake for fifteen minutes.
4. Combine scallion with sour cream in a bowl. Serve the beef casserole hot with a spoonful of the sour cream mixture, green salad, and guacamole

Nutrition:
- Calories: 750.2
- Protein: 48.6g
- Carbs: 7.5g
- Fat: 55.7g
- Fiber: 4.2g

Keto Chicken and Roasted Veggies

Preparation Time: 15 Minutes
Cooking Time: 25 Minutes
Servings: 2

Ingredients:
For the roasted veggies:
- 1/2 pound of Brussels sprouts
- 4 ounces of cherry tomatoes
- 3 ounces of mushrooms
- 1/2 tsp. of salt
- 1/8 tsp. of black pepper (ground)
- ½ tsp. of rosemary (dried)
- 1/8 cup of olive oil

For the chicken:
- 2 chicken breasts
- 1/2 ounce of butter
- 2 ounces of herb butter (to serve)

Directions:
1. Preheat your oven to two hundred degrees Celsius.
2. Arrange the veggies in a greased baking dish. Add rosemary, pepper, and salt—drizzle olive oil from the top. Mix the veggies properly.
3. Bake the vegetables for twenty minutes—heat butter in an iron skillet. Add the chicken breasts. Season with pepper and salt. Fry for five minutes.
4. Serve the fried chicken with a dollop of herb butter on top and roasted veggies by the side.

Nutrition:
- Calories: 1060.3
- Protein: 65.7g
- Carbs: 8.2g
- Fat: 80.3g
- Fiber: 6.1g

Salmon Pie

Preparation Time: 15 Minutes

Cooking Time: 45 Minutes

Servings: 2

Ingredients:	
For the pie crust:	**For the filling:**
• 1/2 cup of almond flour	• 4 ounces of salmon (smoked)
• 2 tbsps. of each	• 1/2 cup of mayonnaise
• Sesame seeds	• 1 large egg
• Coconut flour	• 1 tbsp. of dill (chopped)
• 1/2 tbsp. of ground psyllium husk powder	• 1/4 tsp. of onion powder
• 1/2 tsp. of baking powder	• 1/8 tsp. of black pepper (ground)
• 1 pinch of salt	• 2 ounces of cream cheese
• 1 tbsp. of olive oil	• 2 ounces of cheese (shredded)
• 1 large egg	
• 2 tbsps. of water	

Directions:

1. Preheat your oven at one hundred and seventy degrees Celsius.
2. Place the ingredients for the pie crust in a food processor—pulse for making a firm dough. Use parchment paper for lining a springform pan.
3. Press the prepared dough into the prepared pan. Bake the pie crust for fifteen minutes. Combine all the listed filling ingredients in a large bowl, then add the filling into the crust—Bake for thirty minutes.
4. Let the pie sit for five minutes. Serve warm.

Nutrition:

- Calories: 1046.3
- Protein: 33.4g
- Carbs: 5.8g
- Fat: 98.7g
- Fiber: 7.2g

Keto Falafel

Preparation Time: 15 Minutes   **Cooking Time:** 30 Minutes

Servings: 2

Ingredients:
- 4 ounces of mushrooms (sliced)
- 1/4 cup of each
- Olive oil
- Pumpkin seeds
- Almonds
- 1/2 cup of protein powder
- 1/8 cup of water
- 2 tbsps. of chia seeds
- 1 clove of garlic (minced)
- 1 tbsp. of parsley (chopped)
- 1/2 tsp. of each
- Onion powder
- Salt
- Cumin (ground)
- Coriander seed (ground)
- 1/8 tsp. of black pepper (ground)

Directions:
1. Preheat your oven at one hundred and fifty degrees Celsius.
2. Heat a large frying pan. Add the almonds along with the pumpkin seeds—roast for four minutes.
3. Add the almonds and pumpkin seeds into a food processor. Pulse until a coarse mixture form.
4. Heat oil in the same pan. Add the mushrooms—Cook for three minutes. Add cooked mushrooms and the remaining ingredients to the food processor, then add the remaining olive oil.
5. Shape the prepared mixture into balls of four centimeters. Arrange the falafel balls on a greased baking tray.
6. Bake for twenty minutes. Serve the falafels warm with any side dish.

Nutrition:
- Calories: 570.3
- Protein: 27.5g
- Carbs: 5.2g
- Fat: 47.2g
- Fiber: 9.6g

Ham Croquettes

Preparation Time: 15 Minutes

Cooking Time: 4 Minutes

Servings: 2

Ingredients:
- 1/2 pound of ham (cured, diced)
- 2 large egg whites
- 2 tbsps. of oregano (minced)
- 3 tbsps. of chives (minced)
- 1 tbsp. of cider vinegar
- 1/2 cup of almond flour
- 1 cup of coconut oil

Directions:
1. Pulse ham, oregano, one egg white, chives, and oregano in a food processor. Whisk cider vinegar and egg white.
2. Take a large dish and spread the flour. Make balls from the ham paste using your hands. Dip the balls in the mixture of egg white—coat in the almond flour.
3. Heat oil in a large skillet. Add the croquettes—Fry for four minutes. Serve warm.

Nutrition:
- Calories: 1321.3
- Protein: 30.6g
- Carbs: 2.2g
- Fat: 125.6g
- Fiber: 0.3g

Third Week

Food Plan for the Third Week

Day	Breakfast	Lunch	Dinner
1	Strawberry Rhubarb Pie Smoothie	Keto Croque Monsieur	Grilled Lamb Kebabs and Anchovy Salsa Verde
2	Vanilla Chai Smoothie	Chicken Taco Avocados	Keto Salmon with Tomatoes and Pistachio-Olive Tapenade
3	Cinnamon and Almond Porridge	Keto Quesadillas	Meat Pie
4	Bacon, Mushroom, and Swiss Omelet	No-Bread Italian Subs	Skillet Pizza
5	Maple Cranberry Muffins	Basil Avocado Frail Salad Wraps & Sweet Potato Chips	Low-Carb Lasagna
6	Coco-Cashew Macadamia Muffins	Cauliflower Leek Soup	Keto Pasta and Blue Cheese Sauce
7	Chocolate Protein Pancakes	Low-Calorie Cheesy Broccoli Quiche	Easy 30 Minute Keto Chili

Recipes for Breakfast

Strawberry Rhubarb Pie Smoothie

Preparation Time: 5 Minutes

Cooking Time: 0 Minutes

Servings: 2

Ingredients:
- 1 small stalk rhubarb, sliced
- ¼ cup frozen sliced strawberries
- ¾ cup unsweetened cashew milk
- ½ cup full-fat yogurt, plain
- 1-ounce raw almonds
- ½ teaspoon vanilla extract
- Liquid stevia extract, to taste

Directions:
1. In a blender, add the rhubarb, raspberry, and almond milk.
2. Pulse several times over the ingredients.
3. Stir in the remaining ingredients and blend until smooth.
4. Pour into a big glass, and instantly enjoy it.

Nutrition:
- Calories: 285
- Fat: 20g
- Protein: 11g
- Carbohydrates: 17.5g
- Fiber: 5g
- Net carbs: 12.5g

Vanilla Chai Smoothie

Preparation Time: 5 Minutes

Cooking Time: 0 Minutes

Servings: 2

Ingredients:
- 1 cup unsweetened almond milk
- ½ cup full-fat yogurt, plain
- 1 teaspoon vanilla extract
- ¼ teaspoon ground cinnamon
- ¼ teaspoon ground ginger
- Pinch ground cloves
- Pinch ground cardamom
- Liquid stevia extract, to taste

Directions:
1. In a mixer, add all the ingredients.
2. Pulse several times the ingredients then mix smoothly.
3. Pour into a large glass and fully enjoy it.

Nutrition:
- Calories: 115
- Fat:
- Protein: 5g
- Carbs:
- Fiber: 1g
- Net carbs: 6.5g

Cinnamon Almond Porridge	**Bacon, Mushroom, and Swiss Omelet**

Cinnamon Almond Porridge

Preparation Time: 5 Minutes

Cooking Time: 5 Minutes

Servings: 2

Ingredients:
- 1 tablespoon butter
- 1 tablespoon coconut flour
- 1 large egg, whisked
- 1/8 teaspoon ground cinnamon
- Pinch salt
- ¼ cup canned coconut milk
- 1 tablespoon almond butter

Directions:
1. Melt the butter into a small saucepan over low heat.
2. Whisk the coconut with sugar, egg, cinnamon, and salt.
3. Remove the coconut milk while whisking, and stir in the almond butter until smooth.
4. Simmer over low heat, always stirring until heated through.
5. Spoon, then serve in a bowl.

Nutrition:
- Calories: 470
- Fat: 42g
- Protein: 13g
- Carbohydrate: 15g
- Fiber: 8g
- Net carbohydrate: 7g

Bacon, Mushroom, and Swiss Omelet

Preparation Time: 5 Minutes

Cooking Time: 10 Minutes

Servings: 2

Ingredients:
- 3 large eggs, whisked
- 1 tablespoon heavy cream
- Salt and pepper
- 2 slices uncooked bacon, chopped
- ¼ cup diced mushrooms
- ¼ cup shredded Swiss cheese

Directions:
1. Whisk the eggs together in a small bowl with heavy cream, salt, and pepper.
2. Cook the bacon over medium to high heat in a small skillet.
3. Spoon it in a mug, when the bacon is crisp.
4. Steam the skillet over medium heat, then add the chestnuts.
5. Cook the mushrooms until they smoke, then spoon the bacon into the dish.
6. Heat the skillet with the remaining oil.
7. Pour in the whisked eggs, and cook until the egg's bottom begins to set.
8. To scatter the egg, tilt the saucepan and cook until almost set.
9. Spoon the mixture of bacon and mushroom over half of the omelet, then sprinkle with the cheese and fold over.
10. Let the omelet cook until the eggs have been set, and serve hot.

Nutrition:

• Calories: 475	• Fat: 36g
• Protein: 34g	• Carbohydrates: 4g
• Giber: 0.5g	• Net carbs:

Maple Cranberry Muffins

Preparation Time: 10 Minutes
Cooking Time: 20 Minutes
Servings: 2

Ingredients:
- ¾ cups almond flour
- ¼ cup ground flaxseed
- ¼ cup powdered erythritol
- 1 teaspoon baking powder
- 1/8 teaspoon salt
- 1/3 cup canned coconut milk
- ¼ cup coconut oil, melted
- 2 large eggs
- ½ cup fresh cranberries
- 1 teaspoon maple extract

Directions:
1. Preheat the oven to 350°F, and line a paper liner muffin pan.
2. In a mixing bowl, whisk the almond flour along with the ground flaxseed, erythritol, baking powder, and salt.
3. Whisk coconut milk, coconut oil, eggs, and maple extract together in a separate bowl.
4. Move the wet ingredients to the dry until just full, then fold into the cranberries.
5. Spoon the batter into the prepared pan and bake for 18 to 20 minutes until clean comes out the knife inserted in the center.
6. Cook the muffins in the pan for 5 minutes, then switch onto a cooling rack with wire.

Nutrition:
- Calories: 125
- Fat: 11.5g
- Protein:
- Carbs: 3g
- Fiber: 1.5g
- Carbs: 1.5

Coco-Cashew Macadamia Muffins

Preparation Time: 10 Minutes
Cooking Time: 25 Minutes
Servings: 2

Ingredients:
- 1 ¾ cups almond flour
- 1 cup powdered erythritol
- ¼ cup unsweetened cocoa powder
- 2 teaspoons baking powder
- ¼ teaspoon salt
- ¾ cup cashew butter, melted
- ¾ cup unsweetened almond milk
- 2 large eggs
- ¼ cup chopped macadamia nuts

Directions:
1. Preheat the oven to 350°F and use paper liners to line a muffin pan.
2. In a mixing bowl, whisk the almond flour along with the erythritol, cocoa powder, baking powder, and salt.
3. Whisk the almond milk, the cashew butter, and the eggs together in a separate bowl.
4. Move the wet ingredients to the dry when mixed, then insert them into the nuts.
5. Spoon the batter into the prepared pan and bake for 22 to 25 minutes until clean comes out the knife inserted in the middle.
6. Cook the muffins in the pan for 5 minutes, then switch onto a cooling rack with wire.

Nutrition:
- Calories: 230
- Fat: 20g
- Protein: 9g
- Carbohydrates: 9g
- Fiber: 2.5g
- Net carbs 6.5g

Chocolate Protein Pancakes

Preparation Time: 5 Minutes

Cooking Time: 15 Minutes

Servings: 2

Ingredients:
- 1 cup canned coconut milk
- ¼ cup coconut oil
- 2 large eggs
- 2 scoops (40g) egg white protein powder
- ¼ cup unsweetened cocoa powder
- 1 teaspoon vanilla extract
- Liquid stevia extract, to taste

Directions:
1. In a food processor, add coconut milk, coconut oil, and eggs.
2. Pulse the mixture several times and then add the other ingredients.
3. Mix until smooth and well–change sweetness to taste.
4. Heat medium-heat a non-stick skillet.
5. Using about 1/4 cup per pancake, spoon in batter.
6. Cook until bubbles form at the batter's surface, then flip carefully.
7. Let the pancake cook until it browns on the underside.
8. The leftover batter is moved to a plate to keep warm and repeat.

Nutrition:
- Calories: 455
- Fat: 38.5g
- Protein: 23g
- Carbs: 8g
- Fiber: 3g
- Net carbs: 5g

Recipes for Lunch

Keto Croque Monsieur

Preparation Time: 15 Minutes

Cooking Time: 7 Minutes

Servings: 2

Ingredients:
- 2 eggs
- 25grams grated cheese
- 25grams ham
- 40 ml of cream
- 40 ml mascarpone
- 30grams of butter
- Pepper
- Salt
- Basil leaves

Directions:
1. Beat eggs in a bowl, put salt and pepper.
2. Add the cream, mascarpone, and grated cheese then mix.
3. Melt the butter over medium heat. Adjust the heat to low.
4. Add half of the omelet mixture to the frying pan and then place the slice of ham.
5. Put the rest of the omelet mixture over the ham. Fry within 2-3 minutes over low heat.
6. Then put the omelet back in the frying pan to fry for another 1-2 minutes.
7. Garnish with a few basil leaves. Serve.

Nutrition:
- Calories: 350 kcal
- Protein: 31g
- Fat: 24g
- Fiber: 1g
- Carbohydrates: 2g

Chicken Taco Avocados

Preparation Time: 15 Minutes

Cooking Time: 20 Minutes

Servings: 2

Ingredients:	
For the filling: • 1 c. black beans • 1 c. canned corn • 4-oz. green chilies • 1 c. rotisserie chicken • 1 c. cheddar • 1 package taco seasoning • 2 tbsp. cilantro • 3 ripe avocados	**For the dressing:** • 1 c. ranch dressing • ¼ c. lime juice • 1 tbsp. cilantro • 1 tsp. kosher salt • 1 tsp. ground black pepper

Directions:
1. Warm up the broiler to cook.

For the filling:
1. Mix black beans, corn, 1/2 can of green chilies, shredded chicken, cheddar, taco seasoning, and fresh cilantro in a bowl.
2. Halve three avocados and split, eliminating the pit.
3. Mash the flesh in a small bowl inside, and set aside.
4. Fill the avocado boats with 1/3 cup of filling.
5. Put cheddar and fresher cilantro, then broil within 2 minutes.

Dressing:
1. Mix ranch dressing, lime juice, remaining green chilies, cilantro, salt, and pepper.
2. Fold in mashed avocados.
3. Remove avocado. Serve with dressing and cilantro.

Nutrition:
Calories: 324   Carbohydrates: 16g

Fat: 24g   Protein: 15g

Keto Quesadillas

Preparation Time: 15 Minutes
Cooking Time: 25 Minutes
Servings: 2
Ingredients:

- 1 tbsp. extra-virgin olive oil
- 1 bell pepper
- 1/2 yellow onion
- 1/2 tsp. chili powder
- Kosher salt
- Ground black pepper
- 3 c. Monterey Jack
- 3 c. cheddar
- 4 c. chicken
- 1 avocado
- 1 green onion
- Sour cream

Directions:

1. Warm up the oven to 400°F, and line two medium parchment baking sheets.
2. Warm-up oil in a medium skillet. Put the onion and pepper, chili powder, salt, and pepper. Cook for 5 minutes.
3. Stir cheeses in a medium-sized dish. Put 1 1/2 cups of mixed cheese on the baking sheets. Form a circle, the size of a tortilla flour.
4. Bake the cheeses within 8 to 10 minutes. Put a batter of onion-pepper, shredded chicken, and slices of avocado to one-half each.
5. Cool and fold one side of the tortilla cheese over the side with the fillings. Bake within 3 to 4 more minutes.
6. Serve with green onion and sour cream.

Nutrition:

- Calories: 473
- Carbohydrates: 5g
- Fat: 41g
- Protein: 21g

No-Bread Italian Subs

Preparation Time: 15 Minutes

Cooking Time: 15 Minutes

Servings: 2

Ingredients:

- 1/2 c. mayonnaise
- 2 tbsp. red wine vinegar
- 1 tbsp. extra-virgin olive oil
- 1 small garlic clove, grated
- 1 tsp. Italian seasoning
- 2 slices ham
- 6 salami
- 12 pepperonis
- 1 provolone
- 1 c. romaine
- 1/2 c. roasted red peppers

Directions:

1. For the creamy Italian dressing:
2. Mix the mayo, vinegar, butter, garlic, and Italian seasoning.
3. To assemble sandwiches:
4. Stack a ham slice, two salami pieces, two pepperoni slices, and a provolone slice.
5. Put a handful of romaine and a couple of roasted red peppers.
6. Put creamy Italian sauce, then roll in and eat.

Nutrition:

- Calories: 390
- Protein: 16g
- Carbohydrates: 3g
- Fat: 34g

Basil Avocado Frail Salad Wraps & Sweet Potato Chips

Preparation Time: 15 Minutes

Cooking Time: 30 Minutes

Servings: 2

Ingredients:		
For the sweet potato chips: • Kosher salt • Ground black pepper • Cooking spray • 2-3 medium potatoes	**For the shrimp salad:** • ¼ small red onion • 20 large frails • 1 ½ c. halved grape tomatoes • Cooking spray • 2 avocados • 4 fresh basil leaves • 2 large heads of butterhead lettuce	**For the marinade:** • 2 lemon juice • 2garlic cloves • 3 basil leaves • 2 tbsp. white wine vinegar • 3 tbsp. extra-virgin olive oil • 1/2 tsp. paprika • Kosher salt • Ground black pepper

Directions:
1. For sweet potato chips:
2. Warm up the oven to 375°F then grease a large baking sheet. Put the sweet potato wedges with salt and pepper.
3. Roast within 15 minutes, then flip and roast for 15 minutes. Cool and put aside.
4. For shrimp salad:
5. Grease a large skillet, cook the shrimp, occasionally stirring, within 2 minutes per side. Set aside.
6. For marinade:
7. Mix the lemon juice, garlic, basil, vinegar, butter, and paprika. Put salt and pepper.
8. Stir the tomatoes, onion, avocados, and basil. Fold in the shrimps. Mix.
9. Serve with lettuce cups.

Nutrition:
• Calories: 80
• Carbohydrates: 19g
• Fat: 0g
• Protein: 1g

Cauliflower Leek Soup

Preparation Time: 15 Minutes

Cooking Time: 45 Minutes

Servings: 2

Ingredients:
- ½ tablespoons olive oil
- ½ tablespoon garlic
- ½ tablespoons butter
- 2 cups Vegetable Broth
- 1 leek
- Salt
- 1 cup cauliflower
- Black pepper
- ¼ cup heavy cream

Directions:
1. Heat the oil and butter in the pan.
2. Add garlic, cauliflower, and leek pieces and cook within 5 minutes on low.
3. Add vegetable broth and boil. Cover the pan and cook on low within 45 minutes.
4. Remove then blend the soup in a mixer. Put heavy cream, salt, pepper, and blend more.
5. Serve with salt and pepper.

Nutrition:
- Calories: 155 kcal
- Fats: 13. 1g
- Carbohydrates: 8.3g
- Proteins: 2.4g

Low-Calorie Cheesy Broccoli Quiche

Preparation Time: 2 Minutes

Cooking Time: 30 Minutes

Servings: 2

Ingredients:
- 1/3 tablespoon butter
- Black pepper
- 4 oz. broccoli
- ¼ teaspoon garlic powder
- 2 tablespoon full-fat cream
- 1/8 cup scallions
- Kosher salt
- ¼ cup cheddar cheese
- 2 eggs

Directions:
1. Warm up the oven to 360°F, then grease the baking dish with butter.
2. Put broccoli and 4 to 8 tablespoons of water. Place the bowl in the microwave within 3 minutes.
3. Mix and bake again within 3 minutes.
4. Beat the eggs in a bowl. Pour all leftover items with broccoli.
5. Put all mixture in the baking dish. Bake within 30 minutes.
6. Slice and serve.

Nutrition:
- Calories: 196 kcal
- Fats: 14g
- Carbohydrates: 5g
- Proteins: 12g
- Fiber: 2g

Recipes for Dinner

Grilled Lamb Kebabs and Anchovy Salsa Verde

Preparation Time: 15 Minutes
Cooking Time: 5 Minutes

Servings: 2

Ingredients:	
For the salsa Verde: <ul><li>1/2 cup of each</li><li>Mint</li><li>Parsley</li><li>1 ounce of anchovy (fillets)</li><li>2 tbsps. of each</li><li>Pine nuts</li><li>Capers (drained)</li><li>1 lemon (zested)</li><li>1/4garlic clove</li><li>1/2 tsp. of red pepper flakes</li><li>1 cup of olive oil</li><li>1 pinch of sea salt</li></ul>	**For the lamb kebabs:** <ul><li>8 stems of rosemary</li><li>8 ounces of lamb chops (cut in cubes of one-inch)</li><li>1 eggplant (trimmed, cut into pieces of one-inch)</li><li>Pepper and salt</li><li>1 lemon</li><li>1/4 cup of olive oil</li></ul>

Directions:
1. For the salsa Verde: combine parsley, mint, capers, anchovies, lemon zest, pine nuts, pepper flakes, and garlic in a food processor. While pulsing, add olive oil in a slow stream. Add salt.
2. Heat a grill pan. Remove all the leaves from the rosemary stems, then leave only the top leaves. Chop the leaves.
3. Season the eggplant and lamb with pepper and salt. Sprinkle rosemary on top. Zest the lemon. Add it to the mixture of lamb and eggplant. Add olive oil. Toss for combining.
4. Thread the eggplant and lamb pieces into the rosemary stems, then add the kebab skewers to the grill pan. Grill it for two minutes. Serve the kebabs warms with salsa Verde.

Nutrition:
- Calories: 808.3
- Protein: 15.2g
- Carbs: 6.3g
- Fat: 78.2g
- Fiber: 5.2g

Keto Salmon with Tomatoes and Pistachio-Olive Tapenade

Preparation Time: 15 Minutes

Cooking Time: 15 Minutes

Servings: 2

Ingredients:
- 2 ounces of green olives (pitted)
- 1 1/2 ounce of pistachio nuts (shelled)
- 15 ounces of salmon fillets
- 10 ounces of cherry tomatoes
- 1/2 tbsp. of thyme (dried)
- 1/4 cup of each
- Dill (chopped)
- Olive oil
- Pepper and salt

Directions:
1. Preheat your oven at one hundred and eighty degrees Celsius.
2. Chop the pistachios and olives. Combine them along with a splash of olive oil in a bowl. Arrange the fish's fillets in a large baking dish, then spread the mixture of olives over the fillets.
3. Arrange the tomatoes in another baking dish. Season with thyme, pepper, and salt. Drizzle olive oil on top.
4. Bake the tomatoes and fish for fifteen minutes. Serve the salmon with chopped dill on top and tomatoes by the side.

Nutrition:
- Calories: 840.3
- Protein: 46.7g
- Carbs: 7.6g
- Fat: 66.8g
- Fiber: 5.2g

Meat Pie

Preparation Time: 15 Minutes
Cooking Time: 1 Hour and 5 Minutes

Servings: 2

Ingredients:		
For the pie crust:	**For the topping:**	**For the filling:**
<ul><li>3/4 cup of almond flour</li><li>4 tbsps. of sesame seeds</li><li>5 tbsps. of coconut flour</li><li>1 tbsp. of ground psyllium husk powder</li><li>1/2 tsp. of baking powder</li><li>1 pinch of salt</li><li>3 tbsps. of olive oil</li><li>1 large egg</li><li>5 tbsps. of water</li></ul>	<ul><li>8 ounces of cottage cheese</li><li>7 ounces of cheese (shredded)</li></ul>	<ul><li>1/2 yellow onion (chopped)</li><li>1 clove of garlic (chopped)</li><li>2 tbsps. of butter</li><li>1 pound of beef (ground)</li><li>1 tbsp. of oregano (dried)</li><li>Pepper and salt</li><li>4 tbsps. of tomato paste</li><li>1/2 cup of water</li></ul>

Directions:
1. Preheat your oven at one hundred and seventy degrees Celsius.
2. Heat butter in an iron skillet. Add garlic and onion—Fry for two minutes. Add the beef, then add oregano, pepper, and salt—Fry for five minutes.
3. Add the tomato paste and water. Mix well. Simmer for twenty minutes. Combine all the listed crust ingredients in a food processor.
4. Use parchment paper for lining a springform pan. Add prepared crust in the lined pan, then spread the crust all over the pan. Use your fingers for pressing the crust along the sides.
5. Use a fork for pricking the crust base. Bake the crust for fifteen minutes.
6. Add the beef mixture into the crust. Spread out the filling evenly.
7. Combine cheese and cottage cheese in a bowl. Spread the mixture on top of the meat filling.
8. Bake for forty minutes. Serve warm.

Nutrition:
- Calories: 608.3
- Protein: 35.6g
- Carbs: 6.5g
- Fat: 49.6g
- Fiber: 6.3g

Skillet Pizza

Preparation Time: 15 Minutes

Cooking Time: 5 Minutes

Servings: 2

Ingredients:

- 3 ounces of mozzarella cheese (shredded)
- 2 ounces of sausage (cooked, crumbled)
- 1 ounce of pepperoni slices
- 1 1/2 ounces of green bell pepper (sliced)
- 1/2 tsp. of Italian seasoning
- 2 tbsps. of tomato sauce

Directions:

1. Heat an iron skillet over a medium flame. Sprinkle three-fourths of the cheese on the base of the skillet.
2. Reduce the flame. Top the cheese base with bell pepper, sausage, pepperoni, and remaining cheese—Cook for four minutes.
3. Sprinkle seasoning over the pizza. Remove the skillet from heat. Let the pizza sit for five minutes.
4. Cut the pizza into slices. Serve warm.

Nutrition:

- Calories: 607.6
- Protein: 34.3g
- Carbs: 4.6g
- Fat: 49.9g
- Fiber: 1.2g

Low-Carb Lasagna

Preparation Time: 15 Minutes
Cooking Time: 60 Minutes
Servings: 2
Ingredients:

- 2 tbsps. of olive oil
- 1/2 yellow onion (chopped)
- 2 cloves of garlic (minced)
- 1 pound of Italian sausage
- 1/2 pound of beef (ground)
- 24 ounces of marinara sauce
- 16 ounces of ricotta cheese
- 1 large egg
- 1/2 tsp. of salt
- 1 1/2 pound of deli chicken breast (sliced)
- 3/4 pound of mozzarella cheese (sliced)
- 4 ounces of parmesan cheese

Directions:

1. Preheat your oven at two hundred and twenty degrees Celsius. Heat olive in a frying pan. Add garlic and onion. Fry for three minutes.
2. Add beef and sausage—Cook for five minutes, then add the marinara sauce. Simmer for four minutes. Combine egg, ricotta cheese, and salt in a bowl.
3. For assembling, add half of the meat sauce on the base of a baking dish. Follow with other sliced chicken breast layers, mozzarella cheese, ricotta cheese mixture, and parmesan cheese.
4. Repeat for the remaining ingredients. The top layer will be a layer of parmesan and mozzarella.
5. Cover the dish with aluminum foil—Bake for twenty-five minutes. Remove the foil—Bake for twenty minutes.
6. Let the lasagna sit for fifteen minutes. Serve warm.

Nutrition:

- Calories: 413.6
- Protein: 26.9g
- Carbs: 6.8g
- Fat: 29.5g
- Fiber: 1.3g

Keto Pasta and Blue Cheese Sauce

Preparation Time: 15 Minutes

Cooking Time: 20 Minutes

Servings: 2

Ingredients:		
For the blue cheese sauce: • 7 ounces of each • Cream cheese • Blue cheese • 2 ounces of butter • 2 tsp. of pepper	**For serving:** • 4 tbsps. of pine nuts (roasted) • 2 ounces of parmesan cheese (grated)	**For the pasta:** • 4 large eggs • 5 ounces of cream cheese • 1 tsp. of salt • 3 tbsps. of ground psyllium husk powder

Directions:
1. Preheat your oven at one hundred and fifty degrees Celsius.
2. Mix the cream cheese, eggs, and salt, then add the psyllium husk powder. Let the batter sit for two minutes.
3. Use parchment paper for lining a baking tray. Use a spatula for spreading the batter on the tray. Top with another parchment paper. Flatten the batter using a rolling pin—Bake for twelve minutes.
4. Use a pizza slicer for cutting the pasta into very thin strips. Combine blue cheese along with cream cheese in a saucepan. Stir for five minutes.
5. Add the butter, then warm the sauce for two minutes. Add the pepper. Serve the pasta with blue cheese sauce on top, then garnish with parmesan cheese and pine nuts.

Nutrition:
• Calories: 940.7
• Protein: 35.1g
• Carbs: 8.6g
• Fat: 81.4g
• Fiber: 12.1g

Easy 30 Minute Keto Chili

Preparation Time: 11 Minutes

Cooking Time: 20 Minutes

Servings: 2

Ingredients:
- 32 oz (900g) ground beef (85/15)
- 8 cups spinach
- 1 cup Rao's tomato sauce
- 2 medium green bell peppers
- 2/3 medium onion
- 1 tbsp. olive oil
- 1 tbsp. cumin
- 1 1/2 tbsp. chili powder
- 2 tsp. cayenne pepper
- 1 tsp. garlic powder
- Salt and pepper to taste
- Optional: 1/4 cup parmesan cheese

Directions:
1. Chop the onion and bell peppers into bite-sizes. Sautee in olive oil over medium heat, stirring occasionally.
2. Place the ground beef in a pot over medium-high heat and start to brown it. Once the beef is browned, reduce the heat to low the vegetable, let it cook.
3. Season with salt, pepper, and other spices; whisk to combine. Stir in the spinach, then let it steam for 2-3 minutes, then mix in well.
4. Mix in low carb tomato sauce to the pot, combine well, lower heat to medium-low, and cook for 10 minutes.
5. Mix in the parmesan cheese and then whisk, then pour the vegetables in and whisk again. Cook within a few more minutes, then serve.

Nutrition:
- Calories 467
- Carbs 4.2g
- Fat 30.6g
- Protein 40.1g

Fourth Week

Food Plan for the Fourth Week

Day	Breakfast	Lunch	Dinner
1	Breakfast Roll-Ups	Chicken Curry with Masala	Keto Ham and Broccoli Creamy Casserole
2	Bacon & Avocado Omelet	Cauliflower Mac & Cheese	Chicken Skillet with Jalapeno and Cheese Sauce
3	Bacon & Cheese Frittata	Mushroom & Cauliflower Risotto	Keto Creamy Sun-Dried Tomato Chicken Thighs
4	Bacon & Egg Breakfast Muffins	Pita Pizza	Keto Ground Beef Stroganoff
5	Bacon Hash	Skillet Cabbage Tacos	Keto Salisbury Steak with Mashed Cauliflower
6	Bagels with Cheese	Taco Casserole	Butter Paneer Chicken Curry
7	Baked Apples	Creamy Chicken Salad	Pan-Seared Cod with Tomato Hollandaise

Recipes for Breakfast

Breakfast Roll-Ups

Preparation Time: 5 Minutes

Cooking Time: 15 Minutes

Servings: 2

Ingredients:
- Non-stick cooking spray
- 2 patties of cooked breakfast sausage
- 2 slices of cooked bacon
- 1.5 cups of cheddar cheese, shredded
- Pepper and salt
- 2 large eggs

Directions:
1. Preheat a skillet on medium to high heat, then using a whisk, combine two of the eggs in a mixing bowl.
2. After the pan has become hot, lower the heat to medium-low heat then put in the eggs. If you want to, you can utilize some cooking spray.
3. Season eggs with some pepper and salt.
4. Cover the eggs and leave them to cook for a couple of minutes or until the eggs are almost cooked.
5. Drizzle around 1/3 cup of cheese on top of the eggs, then place a strip of bacon and divide the sausage into two, and place on top.
6. Roll the egg carefully on top of the fillings. The roll-up will almost look like a taquito. If you have a hard time folding over the egg, use a spatula to keep the egg intact until the egg has molded into a roll-up.
7. Put aside the roll-up then repeat the above steps until you have four more roll-ups; you should have 5 roll-ups in total.

Nutrition:
- Calories: 412.2g
- Fats: 31.66g
- Carbohydrates: 2.26g
- Proteins: 28.21g

Bacon & Avocado Omelet

Preparation Time: 5 Minutes

Cooking Time: 5 Minutes

Servings: 2

Ingredients:
- 1 slice crispy bacon
- 2 large organic eggs
- 5 cup freshly grated parmesan cheese
- 2 tbsp ghee or coconut oil or butter
- Half of 1 small avocado

Directions:
1. Prepare the bacon to your liking and set aside. Combine the eggs, parmesan cheese, and your choice of finely chopped herbs. Warm a skillet and add the butter/ghee to melt using the medium-high heat setting. When the pan is hot, whisk and add the eggs.
2. Prepare the omelet working it towards the middle of the pan for about 30 seconds. When firm, flip, and cook it for another 30 seconds. Arrange the omelet on a plate and garnish it with the crunched bacon bits. Serve with sliced avocado.

Nutrition:
- Calories: 719
- Carbohydrates: 3.3grams
- Protein: 30grams
- Fats: 63grams

Bacon & Cheese Frittata	**Bacon & Egg Breakfast Muffins**

Bacon & Cheese Frittata

Preparation Time: 5 Minutes

Cooking Time: 5 Minutes

Servings: 2

Ingredients:
- 1 cup Heavy cream
- 2 Eggs
- 2 Crispy slices of bacon
- 1 Chopped green onion
- 2 oz Cheddar cheese
- Also Needed: 1 pie plate

Directions:
1. Warm the oven temperature to reach 350º Fahrenheit.
2. Whisk the eggs and seasonings. Empty into the pie pan and top off with the remainder of the fixings. Bake 30-35 minutes. Wait for a few minutes before serving for the best results.

Nutrition:
- Carbohydrates: 2grams
- Protein: 13grams
- Fats: 29grams
- Calories: 320

Bacon & Egg Breakfast Muffins

Preparation Time: 15 Minutes

Cooking Time: 30 Minutes

Servings: 2

Ingredients:
- 2 large eggs
- 2 slices bacon
- 1/2 cup green onion

Directions:
1. Warm the oven at 350° Fahrenheit. Spritz the muffin tin wells using a cooking oil spray. Chop the onions and set them aside.
2. Prepare a large skillet using the medium temperature setting. Fry the bacon until it's crispy and place on a layer of paper towels to drain the grease. Chop it into small pieces after it has cooled.
3. Whisk the eggs, bacon, and green onions, mixing well until all of the fixings are incorporated. Dump the egg mixture into the muffin tin (halfway full). Bake it for about 20 to 25 minutes. Cool slightly and serve.

Nutrition:
- Carbohydrates: 0.4grams
- Protein: 5.6grams
- Fats: 4.9grams
- Calories: 69

Bacon Hash	**Bagels with Cheese**
Preparation Time: 5 Minutes	**Preparation Time:** 20 Minutes
Cooking Time: 10 Minutes	**Cooking Time:** 15 Minutes
Servings: 2	**Servings:** 2

Bacon Hash

Preparation Time: 5 Minutes

Cooking Time: 10 Minutes

Servings: 2

Ingredients:
- 1 small green pepper
- 2 jalapenos
- 1 small onion
- 4 eggs
- 6 bacon slices

Directions:
1. Chop the bacon into chunks using a food processor. Set aside for now. Slice the onions and peppers into thin strips. Dice the jalapenos as small as possible.
2. Heat a skillet and fry the veggies. Once browned, combine the fixings and cook until crispy. Place on a serving dish with the eggs.

Nutrition:
- Carbohydrates: 9grams
- Protein: 23grams
- Fats: 24grams
- Calories: 366

Bagels with Cheese

Preparation Time: 20 Minutes

Cooking Time: 15 Minutes

Servings: 2

Ingredients:
- 2.5 cups mozzarella cheese
- 1 tsp. Baking powder
- 3 oz cream cheese
- 1.5 cups almond flour
- 2 eggs

Directions:
1. Shred the mozzarella and combine with the flour, baking powder, and cream cheese in a mixing container. Pop into the microwave for about one minute. Mix well.
2. Let the mixture cool and add the eggs. Break apart into six pieces and shape into round bagels. Note: you can also sprinkle with a seasoning of your choice or pinch of salt if desired.
3. Bake them for approximately 12 to 15 minutes. Serve or cool and store.

Nutrition:
- Carbohydrates: 8grams
- Protein: 19grams
- Fats: 3 1grams
- Calories: 374

Baked Apples

Preparation Time: 10 Minutes

Cooking Time: 60 Minutes

Servings: 2

Ingredients:
- 4 tsp keto-friendly sweetener.
- 2 tsp cinnamon
- .25 cup chopped pecans
- 2 large granny smith apples

Directions:
- Set the oven temperature at 375° Fahrenheit. Mix the sweetener with cinnamon and pecans. Core the apple and add the prepared stuffing.
- Add enough water into the baking dish to cover the bottom of the apple. Bake them for about 45 minutes to 1 hour.

Nutrition:
- Carbohydrates: 16grams
- Protein: 6.8grams
- Fats: 19.9grams
- Calories: 175

Recipes for Lunch

Chicken Curry with Masala

Preparation Time: 15 Minutes
Cooking Time: 30 Minutes

Servings: 2

Ingredients:
- 2 tbsp of oil
- 2 tbsp of minced jalapeño
- 1 ½ pound of diced boneless skinless chicken thighs
- 1 tsp of garam masala
- ¼ cup of chopped cilantro
- 2 tbsp of diced ginger
- 1 cup of chopped tomatoes
- 2 tsp of turmeric
- 1 tsp of cayenne
- 2 tbsp of lemon juice
- 1 tsp of garam masala

Directions:
1. Heat air fryer about 400°F.
2. Grease the air fryer pan with the cooking spray.
3. Add the jalapenos and the ginger.
4. Add in the chicken and the tomatoes then stir.
5. Add the spices, 1 tbsp of oil, 1 tbsp of water.
6. Place the pan in the air fryer and set the temperature to 365°F. Then set the timer to 30 minutes. When the timer beeps, turn off the air fryer.
7. Serve and enjoy your lunch!

Nutrition:
- Calories: 254
- Carbohydrates: 9g
- Protein: 27.8g
- Fats: 14g

Cauliflower Mac & Cheese

Preparation Time: 15 Minutes

Cooking Time: 20 Minutes

Servings: 2

Ingredients:
- 1 head Cauliflower
- 3 tbsp. Butter
- .25 cup Unsweetened almond milk
- .25 cup Heavy cream
- 1 cup Cheddar cheese

Directions:
1. Use a sharp knife to slice the cauliflower into small florets. Shred the cheese. Prepare the oven to reach 450º Fahrenheit. Cover a baking pan with a layer of parchment baking paper or foil.
2. Add two tablespoons of the butter to a pan and melt. Add the florets, butter, salt, and pepper together. Place the cauliflower on the baking pan and roast for 10 to 15 minutes.
3. Warm up the rest of the butter, milk, heavy cream, and cheese in the microwave or double boiler. Pour the cheese over the cauliflower and serve.

Nutrition:
- Net Carbohydrates: 7g
- Protein Counts: 1 1g
- Total Fats: 23g
- Calories: 294g

Mushroom & Cauliflower Risotto

Preparation Time: 5 Minutes

Cooking Time: 10 Minutes

Servings: 2

Ingredients:
- 1grated head of cauliflower
- 1 cup Vegetable stock
- 9 oz. Chopped mushrooms
- 2 tbsp. Butter
- 1 cup Coconut cream

Directions:
1. Pour the stock into a saucepan. Boil and set aside. Prepare a skillet with butter and sauté the mushrooms until golden.
2. Grate and stir in the cauliflower and stock. Simmer and add the cream, cooking until the cauliflower is al dente. Serve.

Nutrition:
- Net Carbohydrates: 4g
- Protein Counts: 1g
- Total Fats: 17g
- Calories: 186

Pita Pizza	**Skillet Cabbage Tacos**
Preparation Time: 15 Minutes	**Preparation Time:** 10 Minutes
Cooking Time: 10 Minutes	**Cooking Time:** 15 Minutes
Servings: 2	**Servings:** 2

Ingredients:

- .5 cup Marinara sauce
- 1 Low-carb pita
- 2 oz.Cheddar cheese
- 14 slices Pepperoni
- 1 oz. Roasted red peppers

Directions:

1. Program the oven temperature setting to 450° Fahrenheit.
2. Slice the pita in half and place it onto a foil-lined baking tray. Rub with a bit of oil and toast for one to two minutes.
3. Pour the sauce over the bread. Sprinkle using the cheese and other toppings. Bake until the cheese melts (5 min.). Cool thoroughly.

Nutrition:

- Net Carbohydrates: 4g
- Protein Counts: 13g
- Total Fats: 19g
- Calories: 250

Ingredients:

- 1 lb. Ground beef
- 5 cup Salsa–ex. Pace Organic
- 2 cups Shredded cabbage
- 2 tsp. Chili powder
- .75 cup Shredded cheese

Directions:

1. Brown the beef and drain the fat. Pour in the salsa, cabbage, and seasoning.
2. Cover and lower the heat. Simmer for 10 to 12 minutes using the medium heat temperature setting.
3. When the cabbage has softened, remove it from the heat and mix in the cheese.
4. Top it off using your favorite toppings, such as green onions or sour cream, and serve.

Nutrition:

- Net Carbohydrates: 4grams
- Protein Counts: 30grams
- Total Fats: 2 1grams
- Calories: 325

Taco Casserole

Preparation Time: 10 Minutes

Cooking Time: 20 Minutes

Servings: 2

Ingredients:
- 1.5 to 2 lb. Ground turkey or beef
- 2 tbsp. Taco seasoning
- 8 oz. Shredded cheddar cheese
- 1 cup Salsa
- .16 oz Cottage cheese

Directions:
1. Heat the oven to reach 400° Fahrenheit.
2. Combine the taco seasoning and ground meat in a casserole dish. Bake it for 20 minutes.
3. Combine the salsa and both kinds of cheese. Set aside for now.
4. Carefully transfer the casserole dish from the oven. Drain away the cooking juices from the meat.
5. Break the meat into small pieces and mash it with a potato masher or fork.
6. Sprinkle with cheese. Bake in the oven for 15 to 20 more minutes until the top is browned.

Nutrition:
- Net Carbohydrates: 6g
- Protein Counts: 45g
- Total Fats: 18g
- Calories: 367

Creamy Chicken Salad

Preparation Time: 10 Minutes
Cooking Time: 30 Minutes
Servings: 2
Ingredients:
- 1 Lb. Chicken Breast
- 2 Avocado
- 2garlic Cloves
- 3 T. Minced Lime Juice
- .33 C. Onion
- 1 Minced Jalapeno Pepper
- 1 T. Minced Salt
- 1 T. Dash Cilantro
- Dash Pepper

Directions:
1. You will want to start this recipe off by prepping the stove to 400°. As this warms up, get out your cooking sheet and line it with paper or foil.
2. Next, it is time to get out the chicken.
3. Go ahead and layer the chicken breast up with some olive oil before seasoning to your liking.
4. When the chicken is all set, you will want to line them along the surface of your cooking sheet and pop it into the oven for about twenty minutes.
5. By the end of twenty minutes, the chicken should be cooked through and can be taken out of the oven for chilling.
6. Once cool enough to handle, you will want to either dice or shred your chicken, dependent upon how you like your chicken salad.
7. Now that your chicken is all cooked, it is time to assemble your salad!
8. You can begin this process by adding everything into a bowl and mashing down the avocado.
9. Once your ingredients are mended to your liking, sprinkle some salt over the top and serve immediately.

Nutrition:
- Fats: 20g
- Carbohydrates: 4g
- Proteins: 25g

Recipes for Dinner

Keto Ham and Broccoli Creamy Casserole

Preparation Time: 15 Minutes

Cooking Time: 45 Minutes

Servings: 2

Ingredients:
- 14 oz (400g) diced ham
- 2 (14-ounce) (800g) bags frozen broccoli
- 8 oz (226g) cream cheese, softened
- 1 cup plain full-fat Greek yogurt
- ½ cup mayonnaise
- 1 tsp garlic salt
- 1 tsp onion powder
- ½ tsp dried basil
- ½ tsp smoked paprika
- ¼ tsp rosemary
- ¼ tsp thyme
- 1 cup shredded cheese
- 1 cup crushed pork rinds

Directions:
1. Prepare to preheat your oven to 350°F (180°C).
2. In a large bowl, add the ham, broccoli, cream cheese, yogurt, mayonnaise, garlic salt, onion powder, basil, smoked paprika, rosemary, and thyme; mix until well combined.
3. Add the casserole mixture into a greased casserole dish. Top with shredded cheese and crushed pork rinds—Bake within 45 minutes or until browned and bubbly.

Nutrition:
- Calories 500
- Carbs 13.6g
- Fat 41.4g
- Protein 42.8g

Chicken Skillet with Jalapeno and Cheese Sauce

Preparation Time: 15 Minutes
Cooking Time: 25 Minutes
Servings: 2

Ingredients:
- 2 tbsp olive oil
- 2 medium chicken thighs
- Salt and pepper, to taste
- ¾ tsp chili powder
- ¾ tsp cumin
- ½ cup onion, finely diced
- 3 medium jalapeños, seeds removed, finely diced
- 2garlic cloves, minced
- ½ cup low-sodium chicken broth
- 4 oz (113g) cream cheese
- 1 cup shredded cheddar cheese

Directions:
1. Prepare to preheat your oven to 425ºF and a large oven-safe skillet over medium-high heat.
2. Add one tbsp of olive oil to the skillet. Rub over the chicken with salt, pepper, chili powder, and cumin.
3. Place the chicken in the skillet and sear on the skin side down for 8-10 minutes. Put the skillet in the oven, then bake within 15 minutes or until cooked through.
4. Remove the chicken thighs and then drain the skillet so that only a few teaspoons of oil remain.
5. Heat the pan over medium-low heat and stir in the onion and jalapenos. Cook for about five minutes, or until softened, add the garlic and cook until fragrant.
6. Mix in the chicken broth and cream cheese. Once it turns into a cream sauce, stir in the shredded cheddar cheese. Place the chicken thighs back in the skillet, serve.

Nutrition:
- Calories 279
- Carbs 3.1g
- Fat 22.1g
- Protein 17.9g

Keto Creamy Sun-Dried Tomato Chicken Thighs

Preparation Time: 15 Minutes
Cooking Time: 15 Minutes
Servings: 2

Ingredients:
Chicken Thighs:
- ½ cup grated Parmesan cheese
- 2-pieces chicken thighs, skinless and boneless
- Salt and pepper, to taste

Creamy Sauce:
- ¼ cup oil from jarred sun-dried tomatoes
- 1 cup drained sun-dried tomatoes, chopped
- 4garlic cloves, minced
- 1 tbsp Italian seasoning
- 1 cup heavy whipping cream
- ¼ cup Parmesan cheese

Directions:
1. Combine the Parmesan cheese, salt, and some pepper on a plate. Coat the chicken in the mixture evenly.
2. Warm the sun-dried tomato oil in a skillet over medium-high heat. Sear the coated chicken for a few minutes on each side, until browned. Set the seared chicken aside.
3. Place the sun-dried tomatoes, garlic, and Italian seasoning in the skillet and cook for a few minutes until the tomatoes start to soften.
4. Put in the heavy cream and the rest of the Parmesan cheese. Combine to create the finished sauce.
5. Add the seared chicken back to the skillet and cook until the chicken is cooked through.

Nutrition:
- Calories 317
- Carbs 8.6g
- Fat 23.6g
- Protein 20.3g

Keto Ground Beef Stroganoff

Preparation Time: 15 Minutes
Cooking Time: 15 Minutes
Servings: 2
Ingredients:

- 2 tbsp butter
- 1 clove minced garlic
- 1 pound 80% lean ground beef
- Salt and pepper, to taste
- 10 oz(228g) sliced mushrooms
- 2 tbsp water
- 1 cup sour cream
- ½ tsp paprika
- 1 tbsp fresh lemon juice
- 1 tbsp fresh chopped parsley

Directions:

1. Put the butter to dissolve in a large skillet over medium heat. When the butter has melted and stops foaming, add the minced garlic to the skillet.
2. Cook the garlic until fragrant, then mix in the ground beef—season with salt and pepper.
3. Cook the ground beef until no longer pink; break up the grounds with a wooden spoon. Remove and set aside in a bowl.
4. Leave only just a little fat in the skillet bottom to cook the mushrooms.
5. Add the mushrooms and water to the pan and cook over medium heat. Cook until the liquid has reduced halfway, and the mushrooms are tender. Set the cooked mushrooms aside.
6. Reduce the heat, then whisk the sour cream and paprika into the skillet. Stir in the cooked beef and mushrooms into the pan and combine. Stir in the lemon juice and parsley.

Nutrition:

- Calories 463
- Carbs 4.1g
- Fat 38.9g
- Protein 23.2g

Keto Salisbury Steak with Mashed Cauliflower

Preparation Time: 15 Minutes
Cooking Time: 30 Minutes
Servings: 2
Ingredients:

- 3 cups cauliflower florets
- 1 tbsp butter & 1 tbsp olive oil
- 3 tbsp unsweetened almond milk
- 12 ounces ground beef
- ¼ cup almond flour
- 2 tsp fresh chopped parsley
- 2 tsp Worcestershire sauce
- ¼ tsp onion powder & ¼ tsp garlic powder
- Salt and pepper, to taste
- 1 ½ cups sliced mushrooms
- ¼ cup beef broth & 2 tbsp sour cream

Directions:

1. Boil the cauliflower in salted water within 5-8 minutes or until tender. Drain the cauliflower, add the butter and almond milk to the cauliflower mash it. Set it aside.
2. Preheat your oven to 375°F (190°C). Line a baking sheet with foil.
3. In a bowl, combine the ground beef, almond flour, parsley, Worcestershire sauce, onion powder, garlic powder, salt, and pepper.
4. Divide the mixture into patties and shape into the Salisbury steaks; put the patties on the foil-lined baking sheet. Bake the patties for 20 minutes or until cooked through.
5. Heat the oil in a large skillet over medium-high heat, add the mushrooms into the skillet, and then cook until they soften and brown.
6. Pour in the beef broth and stir continuously, scraping up and browned bits from the pan's bottom.
7. Stir in the sour cream, then remove the skillet from the heat—season with salt and pepper. Serve with the mashed cauliflower, drizzle with the mushroom gravy.

Nutrition:

- Calories 459
- Carbs 9.4g
- Fat 32.3g
- Protein 34.2g

Butter Paneer Chicken Curry

Preparation Time: 15 Minutes
Cooking Time: 30 Minutes
Servings: 2

Ingredients:

- 2 pounds bone-in chicken thighs
- 7 oz (200g) paneer packet
- 1 cup of water
- 1 cup crushed tomatoes
- ½ cup heavy whipping cream
- 4 tbsp butter
- 1 tbsp olive oil
- 2 tsp coconut oil
- 1 ½ tsp garlic paste
- 1 ½ tsp ginger paste
- 1 tsp coriander powder
- 1 tsp garam masala
- 1 tsp salt
- 1 tsp ground black pepper
- ½ tsp paprika
- ½ tsp Kashmiri Mirch
- ½ tsp red chili powder
- 5 sprigs cilantro

Directions:

1. Preheat oven to 375°F (190°C)
2. Rub chick thighs with olive oil, salt, and pepper to taste. Add the chicken to a baking sheet and roast for 25 minutes.
3. Slice the paneer into small pieces and set aside. Heat the butter and coconut in a pan over medium heat, let the butter start to brown.
4. Mix in the ginger plus garlic paste and sauté for 2 minutes. Add the crushed tomato to the pan.
5. Stir in the coriander powder, garam masala, paprika, red chili powder, and salt. Combine well and allow to simmer until oil shows at the top.
6. Carefully mix the paneer into the sauce. Pour in water and allow it to simmer for 5 minutes.
7. Reduce the heat to medium-low, mix the cream. Stir to combine. Let it simmer until it comes to a boil again. Separate the chicken from the bone.
8. Mix in chicken to the sauce and stir well. Let the curry simmer for at least 5 more minutes. Garnish with cilantro and serve hot.

Nutrition:

- Calories: 819
- Carbs: 3g
- Fat: 67.8g
- Protein: 50.5g

Pan-Seared Cod with Tomato Hollandaise

Preparation Time: 15 Minutes
Cooking Time: 10 Minutes

Servings: 2

Ingredients:	
Pan-Seared Cod: • 1 pound (2-fillets) wild Alaskan Cod • 1 tbsp salted butter • 1 tbsp olive oil	**Tomato Hollandaise:** • 3 large egg yolks • 3 tbsp warm water • 226grams salted butter, melted • 1/4 tsp salt • 1/4 tsp black pepper • 2 tbsp tomato paste • 2 tbsp fresh lemon juice

Directions:
1. Season both sides of the code fillet without salt; the salt will be added in the last. Heat a skillet over medium heat and coat with olive oil and butter.
2. When the butter heats up, place the cod fillet in the skillet and sear on both sides for 2-3 minutes. Baste the fish fillet with the oil and butter mixture.
3. You will know that the cod cooked when it flakes when poked with a fork. Melt the butter in the microwave.
4. In a double boil, beat egg yolks with warm water until thick and creamy and start forming soft peaks. Remove the double boil from the heat, gradually adding the melted butter and stirring.
5. Put salt plus pepper, stir in herbs if desired. Mix in the tomato paste. Stir to combine. Put in the lemon juice, add water to lighten the sauce texture.

Nutrition:
• Calories: 611
• Carbs: 6.9g
• Fat: 52g
• Protein: 25.8g

Fifth Week

Food Plan for the Fifth Week

Day	Breakfast	Lunch	Dinner
1	Tofu Mushrooms	Spicy Keto Chicken Wings	Baked Eggplant Parmesan
2	Spinach Rich Ballet	Sesame-Crusted Tuna with Green Beans	Brussels Sprout and Hamburger Gratin
3	Onion Tofu	Grilled Salmon and Zucchini with Mango Sauce	Lemon Butter Fish
4	Pepperoni Egg Omelet	Slow-Cooker Pot Roast with Green Beans	Chili Lime Cod
5	Nut Porridge	Garlic Chicken	Lemon Garlic Shrimp Pasta
6	Parsley Souffle	Crispy Cuban Pork Roast	One-Pan Tex Mex
7	Eggs and Ham	Keto Barbecued Ribs	Spinach Artichoke-Stuffed Chicken Breasts

Recipes for Breakfast

Tofu Mushrooms

Preparation Time: 5 Minutes

Cooking Time: 10 Minutes

Servings: 2

Ingredients:
- 1 block tofu
- 1 cup mushrooms
- 4 tablespoons butter
- 4 tablespoons parmesan cheese
- Salt
- Ground black pepper

Directions:
1. Toss tofu cubes with melted butter, salt, and black pepper in a mixing bowl.
2. Sauté the tofu within 5 minutes. Stir in cheese and mushrooms.
3. Sauté for another 5 minutes. Serve.

Nutrition:
- Calories: 211
- Total fat: 18.5g
- Cholesterol: 51 mg
- Sodium: 346 mg
- Total carbs: 2g
- Protein: 11.5g

Onion Tofu

Preparation Time: 8 Minutes

Cooking Time: 5 Minutes

Servings: 2

Ingredients:
- 2 blocks tofu
- 2 onions
- 2 tablespoons butter
- 1 cup cheddar cheese
- Salt
- Ground black pepper

Directions:
1. Rub the tofu with salt and pepper in a bowl.
2. Add melted butter and onions to a skillet to sauté within 3 minutes.
3. Toss in tofu and stir cook for 2 minutes. Stir in cheese and cover the skillet for 5 minutes on low heat. Serve.

Nutrition:
- Calories: 184
- Total fat: 12.7g
- Total carbs: 6.3g
- Sugar: 2.7g
- Fiber: 1.6g
- Protein: 12.2g

Spinach Rich Ballet

Preparation Time: 5 Minutes

Cooking Time: 30 Minutes

Servings: 2

Ingredients:
- 3/4 lb. Baby spinach
- 8 teaspoons coconut cream
- 14 oz. Cauliflower
- 2 tablespoons unsalted butter
- Salt
- Ground black pepper

Directions:
1. Warm-up oven at 360 degrees F.
2. Melt butter, then toss in spinach to sauté for 3 minutes.
3. Divide the spinach into four ramekins.
4. Divide cream, cauliflower, salt, and black pepper in the ramekins.
5. Bake within 25 minutes. Serve.

Nutrition:
- Calories: 188
- Total fat: 12.5g
- Cholesterol: 53 mg
- Sodium: 1098 mg
- Total carbs: 4.9g
- Protein: 14.6g

Pepperoni Egg Omelet

Preparation Time: 5 Minutes

Cooking Time: 20 Minutes

Servings: 2

Ingredients:
- 8 pepperonis
- 3 eggs
- 1 tablespoon butter
- 2 tablespoons coconut cream
- Salt and ground black pepper

Directions:
1. Whisk eggs with pepperoni, cream, salt, and black pepper in a bowl.
2. Add ¼ of the butter to a warm-up pan.
3. Now pour ¼ of the batter in this melted butter and cook for 2 minutes on each side. Serve.

Nutrition:
- Calories: 141
- Total fat: 11.3g
- Cholesterol: 181 mg
- Sodium: 334 mg
- Protein: 8.9g

Nut Porridge

Preparation Time: 10 Minutes

Cooking Time: 15 Minutes

Servings: 2

Ingredients:
- 1 cup cashew nuts
- 1 cup pecan
- 2 tablespoons stevia
- 4 teaspoons coconut oil
- 2 cups of water

Directions:
1. Grind the cashews and peanuts in a processor.
2. Stir in stevia, oil, and water. Add the mixture to a saucepan and cook within 5 minutes on high. Adjust on low within 10 minutes. Serve.

Nutrition:
- Calories: 260
- Total fat: 22.9g
- Sodium: 9 mg
- Total carbs: 12.7g
- Sugar: 1.8g
- Fiber: 1.4g
- Protein: 5.6g

Parsley Soufflé

Preparation Time: 5 Minutes

Cooking Time: 6 Minutes

Servings: 2

Ingredients:
- 2 eggs
- 1 red chili pepper
- 2 tablespoons coconut cream
- 1 tablespoon parsley
- Salt

Directions:
1. Blend all the soufflé items into a food processor.
2. Put it in the soufflé dishes, then bake within 6 minutes at 390 degrees f. Serve.

Nutrition:
Calories 108
Total fat 9 g
Cholesterol 180 mg
Sodium 146 mg
Total carbs 1.1 g
Protein 6 g

Eggs and Ham

Preparation Time: 25 Minutes

Cooking Time: 15 Minutes

Servings: 2

Ingredients:
- 2 eggs
- 5 ham slices
- 2 tbsp. of scallions
- A pinch of black pepper
- A pinch of sweet paprika
- 1 tbsp. of melted ghee

Directions:
1. Grease a muffin pan with melted ghee.
2. Divide ham slices of each muffin mold to form your cups. In a bowl; mix eggs with scallions, pepper, and paprika and whisk well.
3. Divide this mix on top of the ham, introduce your ham cups in the oven at 400 °F and bake for 15 minutes.
4. Leave cups to cool down before dividing on plates and serving.

Nutrition:
Calories: 250
Fat: 10 g
Fiber: 3 g
Carbs: 6 g
Protein: 12 g

Recipes for Lunch

Spicy Keto Chicken Wings

Preparation Time: 20 Minutes
Cooking Time: 30 Minutes

Servings: 2

Ingredients:
- Chicken Wings - 2 Lbs.
- Cajun Spice - 1 t.
- Smoked Paprika - 2 t.
- Turmeric - .50 t.
- Salt - Dash
- Baking Powder - 2 t.
- Pepper - Dash

Directions:
1. When you first begin the Ketogenic Diet, you may find that you won't be eating the traditional foods that may have made up a majority of your diet in the past.
2. While this is a good thing for your health, you may feel you are missing out! The good news is that there are delicious alternatives that aren't lacking in flavor! To start this recipe, you'll want to prep the stove to 400.
3. As this heat up, you will want to take some time to dry your chicken wings with a paper towel. This will help remove any excess moisture and get you some nice, crispy wings!
4. When you are all set, take out a mixing bowl and place all of the seasonings along with the baking powder. If you feel like it, you can adjust the seasoning levels however you would like.
5. Once these are set, go ahead and throw the chicken wings in and coat evenly. If you have one, you'll want to place the wings on a wire rack that is placed over your baking tray. If not, you can just lay them across the baking sheet.
6. Now that your chicken wings are set, you are going to pop them into the stove for thirty minutes. By the end of this time, the tops of the wings should be crispy.
7. If they are, take them out from the oven and flip them so that you can bake the other side. You will want to cook these for an additional thirty minutes.
8. Finally, take the tray from the oven and allow it to cool slightly before serving up your spiced keto wings. For additional flavor, serve with any of your favorite, keto-friendly dipping sauce.

Nutrition:
Fats: 7 g
Carbohydrates: 1 g
Proteins: 60 g

Sesame-Crusted Tuna with Green Beans

Preparation Time: 15 Minutes
Cooking Time: 5 Minutes

Servings: 2

Ingredients:

- 1/4 cup white sesame seeds
- 1/4 cup black sesame seeds
- 2 (6-ounce) ahi tuna steaks
- Salt and pepper
- 1 tablespoon olive oil
- 1 tablespoon coconut oil
- 2 cups green beans

Directions:

1. In a shallow dish, mix the two kinds of sesame seeds.
2. Season the tuna with pepper and salt.
3. Dredge the tuna in a mixture of sesame seeds.
4. Heat up to high heat the olive oil in a skillet, then add the tuna.
5. Cook for 1 to 2 minutes until it turns seared, then sear on the other side.
6. Remove the tuna from the skillet, and let the tuna rest while using the coconut oil to heat the skillet.
7. Fry the green beans in the oil for 5 minutes then use sliced tuna to eat.

Nutrition:
380 calories,
19 g fat,
44.5 g protein,
8 g carbs,
3 g fiber,
5 g net carbs

Grilled Salmon and Zucchini with Mango Sauce

Preparation Time: 5 Minutes
Cooking Time: 10 Minutes

Servings: 2

Ingredients:

- 2 (6-ounce) boneless salmon fillets
- 1 tablespoon olive oil
- Salt and pepper
- 1 large zucchini, sliced in coins
- 2 tablespoons fresh lemon juice
- 1/2 cup chopped mango
- 1/4 cup fresh chopped cilantro
- 1 teaspoon lemon zest
- 1/2 cup canned coconut milk

Directions:

1. Preheat a grill pan to heat, and sprinkle with cooking spray liberally.
2. Brush with olive oil to the salmon and season with salt and pepper.
3. Apply lemon juice to the zucchini, and season with salt and pepper.
4. Put the zucchini and salmon fillets on the grill pan.
5. Cook for 5 minutes then turn all over and cook for another 5 minutes.
6. Combine the remaining *Ingredients* in a blender and combine to create a sauce.
7. Serve the side-drizzled salmon filets with mango sauce and zucchini.

Nutrition:
350 calories,
21.5 g of fat,
35 g of protein,
8 g of carbohydrates,
2 g of sugar,
6 g of net carbs

Slow-Cooker Pot Roast with Green Beans

Preparation Time: 10 Minutes
Cooking Time: 8 Hours

Servings: 2

Ingredients:
- 2 medium stalks celery, sliced
- 1 medium yellow onion, chopped
- 1 (3-pound) boneless beef chuck roast
- Salt and pepper
- 1/4 cup beef broth
- 2 tablespoons Worcestershire sauce
- 4 cups green beans, trimmed
- 2 tablespoons cold butter, chopped

Directions:
1. In a slow-cooking dish, add the celery and onion.
2. Put the frying pan on top and season with salt and pepper.
3. Whisk the beef broth and Worcestershire sauce together then pour in.
4. Cover and cook for 8 hours on low heat, until the beef is very tender.
5. Bring the beef off on a cutting board and cut it into chunks.
6. Return the beef to the slow cooker and add the chopped butter and the beans.
7. Cover and cook for 20 to 30 minutes on warm, until the beans are tender.

Nutrition:
375 calories,
13.5 g of fat,
53 g of protein,
6 g of carbohydrates,
2 g of fiber,
4 g of net carbs

Garlic Chicken

Preparation Time: 15 Minutes
Cooking Time: 40 Minutes

Servings: 2

Ingredients:
- Two ounces butter
- Two pounds chicken drumsticks
- Pepper
- salt
- lemon juice
- Two tbsps. olive oil
- Seven cloves garlic
- Half cup parsley

Directions:
1. Warm-up oven at 250 degrees Celsius.
2. Put the chicken in a baking dish. Add pepper and salt.
3. Add olive oil with lemon juice over the chicken. Sprinkle parsley and garlic on top.
4. Bake within forty minutes. Serve.

Nutrition:
Calories: 540.3
Protein: 41.3 g
Carbs: 3.1 g
Fat: 38.6 g
Fiber: 1.6 g

Crispy Cuban Pork Roast

Preparation Time: 15 Minutes

Cooking Time: 4 Minutes

Servings: 2

Ingredients:

- Two pounds pork shoulder
- Four tsp salt
- Two tsp. cumin
- One tsp. black pepper
- Two tbsps. oregano
- One red onion
- Four cloves garlic
- orange juice
- lemons juiced
- One-fourth cup of olive oil

Directions:

1. Rub the pork shoulder with salt in a bowl. Mix all the remaining items of the marinade in a blender.
2. Marinate the meat within eight hours. Cook within forty minutes. Warm-up your oven at 200 degrees. Roast the pork within thirty minutes.
3. Remove the meat juice. Simmer within twenty minutes. Shred the meat.
4. Pour the meat juice. Serve.

Nutrition:
Calories: 910.3
Protein: 58.3 g
Carbs: 5.3 g
Fat: 69.6 g
Fiber: 2.2 g

Keto Barbecued Ribs

Preparation Time: 15 Minutes

Cooking Time: 1 Hour and 10 Minutes

Servings: 2

Ingredients:

- One-fourth cup Dijon mustard
- Two tbsps. of each:
- Cider vinegar
- Butter
- Salt
- Two pounds of spare ribs
- Four tbsps. paprika powder
- Half tbsp. chili powder
- 1&1/2 tbsp. garlic powder
- Two tsp. of each:
- Onion powder
- Cumin
- Two & 1/2 tbsp. black pepper

Directions:

1. Warm-up a grill for thirty minutes.
2. Mix vinegar and Dijon mustard in a bowl, put the ribs, and coat.
3. Mix all the listed spices. Rub the mix all over the ribs. Put aside. Put ribs on an aluminum foil. Add some butter over the ribs. Wrap with foil. Grill within one hour. Remove and slice.
4. Put the reserved spice mix. Grill again within ten minutes. Serve.

Nutrition:
Calories: 980.3
Protein: 54.3 g
Carbs: 5.8 g
Fat: 80.2 g
Fiber: 4.6 g

Recipes for Dinner

Baked Eggplant Parmesan

Preparation Time: 15 Minutes

Cooking Time: 40 Minutes

Servings: 2

Ingredients:
- 1 large eggplant, sliced into 8 1/2"
- sprinkle of salt
- 1 large egg
- ½ cup Parmesan cheese, grated
- ¼ cup ground pork rinds
- ½ tablespoon Italian seasoning
- 1 cup Rao's Arrabbiata Sauce
- ½ cup shredded mozzarella cheese
- 4 tablespoons butter melted

Directions:
1. Prepare to preheat the oven to 400 °F (200 °C). Place the eggplant slice on a baking sheet lined with baking paper and sprinkle both sides with salt. Let sit for at least 30 minutes to allow the water out.
2. Mix the ground pork rinds, parmesan cheese, and Italian seasoning in a shallow bowl. Set aside.
3. Mix the egg in a separate shallow bowl. Add the melted butter to the bottom of a 9x13 inch baking dish.
4. Pat, the eggplant dry with a kitchen towel, set aside. Dip each slice of the eggplant into the beaten egg and then into the parmesan cheese mixture, covering each side with crumbs. Place the eggplant into the butter-coated baking dish.
5. Bake the eggplants for 20 minutes. Turn the pieces over and bake an additional 20 minutes or until golden brown.
6. Pout the marinara sauce over the eggplant and sprinkle with mozzarella cheese.
7. Place the baking sheet bake in the oven for an additional 5 minutes or until the cheese has melted.

Nutrition:
Calories: 313
Carbs: 6.3 g
Fat: 25.7 g
Protein: 11.5 g

Brussels Sprout and Hamburger Gratin

Preparation Time: 15 Minutes

Cooking Time: 20 Minutes

Servings: 2

Ingredients:
- Ground beef, one pound
- Bacon, eight ounces, diced small
- Brussel sprouts, fifteen ounces, cut in half
- Salt, one teaspoon
- Black pepper; one teaspoon
- Thyme; one-half teaspoon
- Cheddar; cheese shredded one cup
- Italian seasoning; one tablespoon
- Sour cream; four tablespoons
- Butter; two tablespoons

Directions:
1. Heat the oven to 425.
2. Fry bacon and Brussel sprouts in butter for five minutes.
3. Stir in the sour paste and pour this mix into a greased eight by the eight-inch baking pan.
4. Cook the ground food and season with salt and pepper, then add this mix to the baking pan.
5. Top with the herbs and the shredded cheese. Bake for twenty minutes.

Nutrition:
Calories: 770 kcal
Net carbs: 8 g
Fat: 62 g
Protein: 42 g

Lemon Butter Fish

Preparation Time: 10 Minutes

Cooking Time: 20 Minutes

Servings: 2

Ingredients:
- 1 tbsp. lemon juice
- 4 tbsp. butter, unsalted
- Sea salt & pepper, to taste
- 2 tbsp. almond flour
- 2 tbsp. olive oil
- 2 tilapia fillets
- Sea salt & pepper, to taste

Directions:
1. Warm the butter in a small pan over medium heat. Warm the butter until it's slightly browned.
2. Add the lemon juice, pepper, and salt and stir constantly. Adjust seasoning to taste. Set aside while you cook your fillets.
3. Rinse the fish fillets and pat them dry before sprinkling them with salt and pepper.
4. Spread the flour on a plate or shallow dish and dredge the fillets, spreading the flour over the fillets as needed.
5. Heat a non-stick skillet over medium heat and warm the oil in it until it's shimmering.
6. Place the fillets in the pan and cook for about two minutes per side until golden and crisp on either side.
7. Remove the fish from the heat and place it on the plate. Drizzle the sauce over it and serve immediately!

Nutrition:
Calories: 393
Fat: 28 g
Carbohydrates: 3 g
Protein: 31 g

Chili Lime Cod

Preparation Time: 10 Minutes
Cooking Time: 10 Minutes

Servings: 2

Ingredients:
- 1/3 c. coconut flour
- 1/2 tsp. cayenne pepper
- 1 egg, beaten
- 1 lime
- 1 tsp. crushed red pepper flakes
- 1 tsp. garlic powder
- 12 oz. cod fillets
- Sea salt & pepper, to taste

Directions:
1. Preheat the oven to 400° Fahrenheit and line a baking sheet with non-stick foil.
2. Place the flour in a shallow dish (a plate works fine) and drag the fillets of cod through the beaten egg. Dredge the cod in the coconut flour, then lay it on the baking sheet.
3. Sprinkle the tops of the fillets with seasoning and lime juice.
4. Bake for 10 to 12 minutes until the fillets are flaky.
5. Serve immediately!

Nutrition:
Calories: 215
Fat: 5 g
Carbohydrates: 3 g
Protein: 37 g

Lemon Garlic Shrimp Pasta

Preparation Time: 10 Minutes
Cooking Time: 10 Minutes

Servings: 2

Ingredients:
- 1/2 lemon, thinly sliced
- 1/2 tsp. paprika
- 1 lb. lg. shrimp, deveined & peeled
- 1 tsp. basil, fresh & chopped
- 7 oz. Miracle Noodle Angel Hair pasta
- 2 cloves garlic, minced
- 2 tbsp. butter
- 2 tbsp. extra virgin olive oil
- Sea salt & pepper, to taste

Directions:
1. Drain the packages of Miracle noodles and rinse them under cool running water.
2. Bring a pot of water to a boil and place the noodles in the boiling water for two minutes before pulling them back out again.
3. Place the boiled noodles in a hot pan over medium heat and allow the excess moisture to cook off of them. Set aside.
4. Add the butter and olive oil to the pan, then add the garlic and stir.
5. Place the shrimp and the lemon slices in the pan and allow to cook until the shrimp is done, about three minutes per side.
6. Once the shrimp is done, add the salt, pepper, and paprika to the pan, then top with the noodles.
7. Toss to coat everything together, top with basil, and serve!

Nutrition:
Calories: 360
Fat: 21 g
Carbohydrates: 4 g
Protein: 36 g

One-Pan Tex Mex

Preparation Time: 5 Minutes
Cooking Time: 10 Minutes
Servings: 2

Ingredients:

- 1/3 c. baby corn, canned
- 1/3 c. cilantro, chopped & separated
- 1/2 c. chicken stock
- 1/2 c. diced tomatoes & green chiles
- 1/2 tsp. garlic powder
- 1/2 tsp. oregano
- 1 tsp. cumin
- 2 c. cauliflower, riced
- 2 c. chicken breast, cooked & diced
- 2 c. Mexican cheese blend, shredded
- 2 tbsp. extra virgin olive oil
- 2 tsp. chili powder

Directions:

1. Slice baby corn into small pieces and set aside. Press any liquid out of the riced cauliflower and set aside.
2. In a large pan over medium heat, warm your oil and sauté the cauliflower rice for about two minutes.
3. Add all ingredients except for the cheese and cilantro, and stir well to cook.
4. Stir in about half of the cilantro and allow the flavors to meld.
5. Stir about half the cheese into the mix and stir until melted and combined.
6. Serve and top with remaining cheese and cilantro for garnish!

Nutrition:
Calories: 345
Fat: 26 g
Carbohydrates: 7 g
Protein: 38 g

Spinach Artichoke-Stuffed Chicken Breasts

Preparation Time: 15 Minutes
Cooking Time: 15 Minutes
Servings: 2

Ingredients:

- 1/4 c. Greek yogurt
- 1/4 c. spinach, thawed & drained
- 1/2 c. artichoke hearts, thinly sliced
- 1/2 c. mozzarella cheese, shredded
- 1/2 lb. chicken breasts
- 2 tbsp. olive oil
- 4 oz. cream cheese
- Sea salt & pepper, to taste

Directions:

1. Pound the chicken breasts to a thickness of about one inch. Using a sharp knife, slice a "pocket" into the side of each. This is where you will put the filling.
2. Sprinkle the breasts with salt and pepper and set aside.
3. In a medium bowl, combine cream cheese, yogurt, mozzarella, spinach, artichoke, salt, and pepper and mix completely. A hand mixer may be the easiest way to thoroughly combine all the ingredients.
4. Spoon the mixture into the pockets of each breast and set aside while you heat a large skillet over medium heat and warm the oil in it. If you have an extra filling you can't fit into the breasts, set it aside until just before your chicken is done cooking.
5. Cook each breast for about eight minutes per side, and then pull off the heat when it reaches an internal temperature of about 165° Fahrenheit.
6. Just before you pull the chicken out of the pan, heat the remaining filling to warm it through and to rid it of any cross-contamination from the chicken. Once hot, top the chicken breasts with it.
7. Serve!

Nutrition:

Calories: 288	Fat: 17 g
Carbohydrates: 2 g	Protein: 28 g

Chapter 15: Other Recipes

Chocolate Cheesecake

Preparation Time: 10 Minutes   **Cooking Time:** 2 Hours

Servings: 2

Ingredients:
- 1/4 cup almond flour
- 1/4 cup cocoa powder
- 1/4 cup Swerve sweetener
- 3 tablespoons melted vegan butter
- 3 ounces dark chocolate
- 1 tablespoon vegan butter
- 6 ounces cream cheese
- 1/2 cup Swerve sweetener
- Sweetener with 1 cup of powder
- 1 tablespoon vanilla extract
- 2 large eggs
- 1/4 cup cocoa powder
- 1/3 cup thick cream
- 2 teaspoons melted butter
- 3/4 fresh cane
- 3 oz. chopped chocolate
- 1/2 teaspoon vanilla extract

Directions:
1. Preheat oven to 325F. Mix the almond flour, cocoa powder, and sweetener. Stir in the melted butter.
2. Press the mixture well into the bottom of a 9-inch bow-shaped container. Bake 10 minutes, then remove and reduce oven temperature to 300F.
3. In a small saucepan over medium heat, mix the dark chocolate with butter. Set aside.
4. Beat cream cheese, sweeteners and vanilla extract, then eggs one by one, scraping the sides and sides of the bowl.
5. Mix cocoa powder and thick cream, then add melted chocolate.
6. Grease with melted butter, don't disturb the crust. Put filling into the pan and shake gently.
7. Bake 60 minutes. Remove and let cool completely. After cooling, remove the sides, cover well in plastic wrap and refrigerate for at least 3 hours.
8. Over medium heat, incorporate cream and the sweetener. Simmer, put off heat and add chopped chocolate and vanilla. Set aside and then beat until smooth.
9. Pour over the top of cold cheese.

Nutrition:
Fat: 32.98 g   Protein: 7.75 g   Carbohydrates: 5.22 g

Walnut Bites

Preparation Time: 15 Minutes

Cooking Time: 0 Minutes

Servings: 2

Ingredients:

- 1 ½ cup Old Fashioned oats
- 3 tablespoons dark cocoa
- ½ teaspoon cinnamon
- 1 cup pitted soft dates
- 3 tablespoons almond butter
- 3 tablespoons dark pure maple syrup
- 3 tablespoons chopped walnuts
- 3 tablespoons mini chocolate chips

Directions:

1. Crush the oatmeal. Transfer in a bowl. Mix cocoa, cinnamon, and salt.
2. Crush dates then add almond butter and maple syrup to make a thick paste.
3. Mold the dough to the silicone to begin to resemble crushed cookie dough, about 2 minutes. Continue the work on the dough.
4. Mix nuts and chocolate chips. Knead well.
5. Form into 14 balls.
6. Refrigerate the refrigerator to adjust the chocolate.

Nutrition:
Fat: 4 g
Carbohydrates: 5 g
Protein: 2 g

Cinnamon Pudding

Preparation Time: 10 Minutes

Cooking Time: 60 Minutes

Servings: 2

Ingredients:

- 3 eggs
- 3/4 cup thick cream
- 1/2 splendid cane
- 1/4 cup unsweetened caramel topping
- 1 cup almond flour
- 1/4 teaspoon baking powder
- 1 cup cottage cheese
- 1/4 teaspoon cinnamon

Directions:

1. Beat all the ingredients with the mixer
2. Pour into an 8x8 "glass baking dish with butter and sprinkle extra cinnamon.
3. Bake at 350 ° F for 1 hour.

Nutrition:
Fat: 18 g
Protein: 2 g
Carbohydrates: 8 g

Cheesecake Mousse

Preparation Time: 5 Minutes

Cooking Time: 0 Minutes

Servings: 2

Ingredients:
- 8 ounces softened cream cheese
- 1/3 cup erythritol powder
- 1/8 teaspoon concentrated stevia powder
- 1 1/2 teaspoons vanilla extract
- 1/4 teaspoon lemon extract
- 1 cup thick whipped cream

Directions:
1. Beat the cream cheese until smooth.
2. Mix the extract of erythritol, stevia, vanilla, and lemon.
3. Beat the thick cream with the mixer until stiff peaks form.
4. Fold half the whisk in the cream cheese mixture. Fold the other half of the whip.
5. Beat until it is soft and fluffy.
6. In the refrigerator for 2 hours.
7. Melt with fresh fruit.

Nutrition:
27.8 g fat
3.7 g protein
16.5 g carbohydrates

No-Crust Pumpkin Pie

Preparation Time: 10 Minutes

Cooking Time: 40 Minutes

Servings: 2

Ingredients:
- 2 tablespoons butter
- 4 tablespoons coconut without sugar
- 6 oz. pumpkin
- 2/3 heavy fresh cane
- 1-ounce butter
- 2 teaspoons pumpkin pie
- 1 teaspoon baking powder
- 2 eggs
- 1/4 cups thick cream

Directions:
1. Chop squash into cubes and position it in a pan. Boil wheat, butter, and salt over medium heat.
2. Simmer for 20 minutes. Stir occasionally.
3. Once it is soft, mix the remaining ingredients, except the eggs with a hand blender.
4. Whisk eggs with a hand mixer for 3 minutes. Add the purified pumpkin and mix.
5. Prep oven to 400 ° F. Grease a 9 "baking dish with butter and apply the coconut flakes evenly.
6. Bake for 20 minutes.

Nutrition:
10 g fat
2 g protein
2 g carbohydrates

Coconut Blondies

Preparation Time: 5 Minutes

Cooking Time: 20 Minutes

Servings: 2

Ingredients:
- 1/2 cup untreated butter
- 1/2 cup erythritol
- 4 eggs
- 1/2 cup coconut flour
- 1/4 cup coconut milk
- 1/2 cup unsweetened coconut
- 1 tablespoon vanilla extract
- 1/4 teaspoon baking powder
- 1/4 teaspoon salt

Directions:
1. Preheat oven to 350F degrees
2. Grease and line an 8-inch baking sheet with parchment paper.
3. Mix the butter and erythritol until smooth.
4. Stir eggs.
5. Beat vanilla extract and coconut milk.
6. Then mix coconut flour, dried coconut, baking powder, and salt.
7. Position the baking sheet and bake for 30 minutes.
8. Set aside for 30 minutes.

Nutrition:
17 g fat
4 g protein
6 g carbohydrates

Italian Crackers

Preparation Time: 10 Minutes

Cooking Time: 15 Minutes

Servings: 2

Ingredients:
- 1/ 2 Almond flour
- 2 teaspoons olive oil
- 3/4 teaspoon salt
- 1/4 tablespoon basil
- 1/2 teaspoon thyme
- 1/4 teaspoon oregano
- 1/2 tablespoon onion powder
- 1/4 teaspoon Garlic powder

Directions:
1. Preheat oven to 350 degrees F.
2. Incorporate all the ingredients to create a dough.
3. Form the dough into a long rectangular log and then cut it into thin slices ½ cm thick. Position on a baking sheet with parchment paper.
4. Bake 12 minutes.

Nutrition:
90 calories
10 g fats
7 g carbohydrates

Keto Barueri Cocoa

Preparation Time: 5 Minutes

Cooking Time: 20 Minutes

Servings: 2

Ingredients:
- Coconut layer:
- 2 cups shredded coconut
- 1/3 c of coconut oil
- 1/4 cup granulated concealer
- Chocolate cover layer:
- 3 squares of Baker's unsweetened chocolate
- 1 tablespoon coconut oil
- 1-2 tablespoons nutritive sweetener

Directions:
1. Coconut layer.
2. Blend coconut, coconut oil, and sweetener into a food processor with the S blade.
3. Mash down the coconut mixture into the bottom of a silicone pan.
4. Freeze while preparing the cover.
5. Chocolate coating
6. Heat coconut oil and chocolate to 50% microwave power until melted.
7. Add the sweetener if you use unsweetened chocolate.
8. Spread evenly over the frozen coconut layer. Chill for 30 minutes.
9. Remove the freezer.
10. Rotate the silicone molds inward to release the frozen content.

Nutrition:
22 g fat
11 g protein
4 g carbohydrates

Baked Granola

Preparation Time: 5 Minutes

Cooking Time: 20 Minutes

Servings: 2

Ingredients:
- 1/2 cup canola oil
- 1/2 cup honey
- 1/2 tsp. cinnamon
- 1/2 tsp. salt
- 3 cups old-fashioned rolled oats
- 1 cup almonds
- 1 cup raisins

Directions:
1. Ready oven to 300 degrees F and glues a baking sheet with parchment paper. Fix a shelf in the middle of the oven.
2. Sprinkle a baking sheet with anchovy paper.
3. Reserve
4. Mix the oil, honey, cinnamon, and salt. Put the oil, honey, cinnamon, and salt.
5. Add oats and almonds and stir. Stir in barley and almonds directly in the oil mixture.
6. Spread the oatmeal on the ready baking sheet. Use a spatula to press it into the pot.
7. Bake for 20 minutes, stirring halfway.
8. Bake, stir for about half a minute, about 20 minutes.
9. Remove from the oven.
10. Place on a wire rack and sprinkle the raisins or nuts.
11. Cool completely before storing it.

Nutrition:
5 g Carbohydrates
12 g Protein
16 g Fat

Protein Power Sweet Potatoes

Preparation Time: 5 Minutes

Cooking Time: 45 Minutes

Servings: 2

Ingredients:
- 2 medium sweet potatoes
- 6 ounces plain Greek yogurt
- ½ teaspoon salt
- 1/3 cup dried cranberries
- ¼ teaspoon black pepper

Directions:
1. Heat the oven to 400 degrees F and prick sweet potatoes several times.
2. Place them on a cooking plate and cook for 45 minutes.
3. Cut the potatoes in half and wrap the meat in a medium bowl and keep the skin healthy.
4. Mix the salt, pepper, yogurt, and cranberries.
5. Scoop the mix into the potato skins and serve warm.

Nutrition:
11 g Fat
15 g Carbohydrates
18 g Protein

Penne Pasta with Vegetables

Preparation Time: 10 Minutes

Cooking Time: 5 Minutes

Servings: 2

Ingredients:
- 1 teaspoon salt
- ¾ cup uncooked penne pasta
- 1 tablespoon olive oil
- 1 tablespoon garlic
- 1 teaspoon fresh oregano
- 1 cup mushrooms
- 2 cherry tomatoes
- l cup fresh spinach leaves
- ½ teaspoon black pepper
- 1 tablespoon Parmesan cheese

Directions:
1. Boil 1-quart water to a boil. Sprinkle 1/2 teaspoon of the salt and the penne, and cook according to package directions. Drain but do not rinse the penne, reserving about VA cup pasta water.
2. Heat the olive oil over medium-high heat. Sauté the garlic, oregano, and mushrooms for 5 minutes.
3. Sauté the tomatoes and seasoned spinach for 4 minutes.
4. Situate drained pasta to the skillet, along with 3 tablespoons of the pasta water. Cook, constantly stirring, for 3 minutes.
5. Sprinkle with Parmesan cheese.
6. Serve.

Nutrition:
12 g Fat
9 g Carbohydrates
19 g Protein

Cinnamon and Spice Overnight Oats

Preparation Time: 10 Minutes

Cooking Time: 0 Minutes

Servings: 2

Ingredients:

- 75 g rolled oats
- 100 ml milk
- 75 g yogurt
- 1 tsp. honey
- 1/2 tsp. vanilla extract
- 1/8th tsp. Schwartz ground cinnamon
- 20 g raisins

Directions:

1. Mix all ingredients.
2. Cover overnight or at least one hour and refrigerate.
3. Exit the refrigerator or heat it in the microwave immediately or slowly.
4. Serve and enjoy.

Nutrition:

15 g Carbohydrates

26 g Protein

34 g Fat

Cheese Stuffed Mushrooms

Preparation Time: 10 Minutes

Cooking Time: 15 Minutes

Servings: 2

Ingredients:

- 2 large mushrooms, clean, remove stems and chopped stems finely
- 1 ½ tbsp fresh parsley, chopped
- 1 garlic clove, minced
- ½ cup parmesan cheese, grated
- ¼ cup Swiss cheese, grated
- 3.5 oz cream cheese
- 1 tbsp olive oil
- Salt

Directions:

1. Preheat the oven to 375 degrees.
2. Toss mushrooms with olive oil and place them onto a baking tray. In a bowl, combine cream cheese, chopped mushrooms stems, parsley, garlic, parmesan cheese, Swiss cheese, and salt.
3. Stuff cream cheese mixture into the mushroom caps and arrange mushrooms on the baking tray. Bake in preheated oven for 10-15 minutes.
4. Serve and enjoy.

Nutrition:

79 Calories

6.3 g Fat

4 g Protein

Delicious Chicken Alfredo Dip

Preparation Time: 10 Minutes
Cooking Time: 20 Minutes

Servings: 2

Ingredients:

- 1 cup chicken, cooked and chopped into small pieces
- 1 ½ tbsp fresh parsley, chopped
- 1 tomato, diced
- 2 bacon slices, cooked and crumbled
- 1 ½ cups mozzarella cheese, shredded
- 1 tsp Italian seasoning
- ½ cup parmesan cheese, grated
- 2 oz cream cheese, softened
- 1 ½ cups Alfredo sauce, homemade & low-carb

Directions:

1. Preheat the oven to 375 degrees.
2. Put some cooking spray on the baking dish and set it aside.
3. Add chicken, ½ cup mozzarella cheese, Italian seasoning, parmesan cheese, cream cheese, and Alfredo sauce to the bowl and stir to combine.
4. Spread chicken mixture into the prepared baking dish and top with remaining mozzarella cheese.
5. Bake in preheated oven for 20 minutes.
6. Top with parsley, tomatoes, and bacon. Serve and enjoy.

Nutrition:
Calories: 144   Fat : 0.5 g   Protein: 29.3 g

Guacamole

Preparation Time: 10 Minutes

Cooking Time: 5 Minutes

Servings: 2

Ingredients:

- 2 avocados, halved and pitted
- 1 tbsp fresh lemon juice
- 2 garlic cloves, minced
- ¼ tsp ground cumin
- 2 tbsp fresh parsley, chopped
- ½ jalapeno pepper, chopped
- 2 tbsp onion, chopped
- ½ tsp sea salt

Directions:

1. Scoop out avocado's flesh using a spoon and place it into the bowl.
2. Mash the avocado flesh using a fork. Combine the remaining ingredients.
3. Serve and enjoy.

Nutrition:
106 Calories
9.9 g Fat
1.1 g Protein

Perfect Cucumber Salsa	Chocolate Chip Cookie
Preparation Time: 5 Minutes	**Preparation Time:** 15 Minutes
Cooking Time: 5 Minutes	**Cooking Time:** 1 Minute
Servings: 2	**Servings:** 2

Perfect Cucumber Salsa

Ingredients:
- 1 cup cucumbers, peeled, seeded, and chopped
- 1 tsp fresh cilantro, chopped
- 1 tsp fresh parsley, chopped
- ½ tbsp fresh lemon juice
- 1 garlic clove, minced
- 1 small onion, chopped
- 1 large jalapeno pepper, chopped
- ½ cup tomatoes, chopped
- ½ tsp salt

Directions:
1. Mix all ingredients into the large mixing bowl until well combined.
2. Serve and enjoy.

Nutrition:
14 Calories
0.2 g Fat
0.6 g Protein

Chocolate Chip Cookie

Ingredients:
- Balls
- 1 cup almond flour
- ½ teaspoon vanilla extract
- 1 tablespoon powdered swerve sweetener
- ¼ cup dark chocolate chips
- ¼ cup heavy cream
- Chocolate Ganache
- 1 ½ tablespoon dark chocolate
- 1 tablespoon unsalted butter

Directions:
1. Mix flour in it, add vanilla, sweetener, and cream.
2. Fold in chocolate chips, and shape the mixture into balls.
3. Melt chocolate and butter in the microwave for 1 minute, stir every 15 seconds.
4. Drizzle chocolate over the balls, rest for 5 minutes, and serve.

Nutrition:
74 Calories
7 g Fat
2 g Protein

Cream Cheese Fudge	Blueberry Ice Pops
Preparation Time: 4 Hours	**Preparation Time:** 5 Minutes
Cooking Time: 2 Minutes	**Cooking Time:** 20 Minutes
Servings: 2	**Servings:** 2

Cream Cheese Fudge

Ingredients:

- 2 ounces chocolate
- ½ cup powdered stevia
- 1 tablespoon vanilla extract
- ½ cup salted butter
- 8 ounces cream cheese, full-fat

Directions:

1. Melt chocolate and butter for 2 minutes stir every 30 seconds.
2. Whisk sweetener and vanilla using an electric blender
3. Mix cream cheese in it, pour in chocolate mixture, using a hand whisk.
4. Take a 6-by-8-inch pan, grease it with oil, spoon the chocolate mixture, and spread evenly.
5. Freeze 4 hours, then cut and serve.

Nutrition:
145 Calories
13.6 g Fat
2.9 g Protein

Blueberry Ice Pops

Ingredients:

- 3 ounces fresh blueberries
- 35 drops of liquid stevia
- 1 tablespoon lemon juice
- 1 cup coconut milk

Directions:

1. Blend all the ingredients in the food processor.
2. Pour the mixture into ice pop molds and freeze for 6 hours.
3. Dip each pop mold into hot water to release.

Nutrition:
154 Calories
15.2 g Fat
3.2 g Protein

Blueberry Crisp

Preparation Time: 5 Minutes

Cooking Time: 20 Minutes

Servings: 2

Ingredients:
- 1/8 cup almond flour
- 1 cup fresh blueberries
- 2 tablespoons powdered swerve sweetener
- ¼ cup pecan halves
- 1 tablespoon ground flax
- ¼ teaspoon salt
- ½ teaspoon ground cinnamon
- ½ teaspoon vanilla extract
- 2 tablespoons unsalted butter
- 2 tablespoons heavy cream

Directions:
1. Preheat oven to 400°F.
2. Fill each ramekin with ½ cup berries and ½ tablespoon sweetener, and stir.
3. Blend remaining ingredients into a food processor, spoon this mixture over berries.
4. Bake for 20 minutes, top each with 1 tablespoon of heavy cream.

Nutrition:
390 Calories
35 g Fat
6 g Protein

Conclusion

I hope this book was able to help you have a better understanding about the keto lifestyle and how the diet works. In truth, the Ketogenic diet is considered to be one of the most effective and popular diets of today. Apart from its popularity, this diet also offers tremendous health benefits to the body.

The keto diet is a meal plan that allows your body to produce ketones and then go into a state of ketosis. Ketones are produced when the body uses fat as the source of energy instead of glucose. This is possible because the diet consists of meals that reduce the intake of sugars and carbohydrates, thus depleting the glucose storage in the body. This is the reason why people are able to lose weight and keep it off when following this diet.

However, loss of weight is not the only benefit of following this diet. People are also able to treat ailments such as epilepsy and also prevent certain lifestyle diseases such as Type I and Type II diabetes. Even though there are some side effects that persons may encounter when they just begin the diet, they do not only alleviate them through applying the suggestions deliberated in the book, but the permanent advantages far outweigh their temporary effects. The diet is very simple and easy to follow and can fit into your lifestyle.

Diabetes can be an annoying condition with lots of limitations and risks, however, it doesn't have to be a life sentence. Awareness is the first step to making conscious change. The next step is to be determined to make a conscious change. Develop a plan and jump into action. There are several things that you can do in order to control diabetes, the most important and perhaps the most powerful one of them is modifying your dietary habits. We hope that you have found our guidance on low carb foods, foods to seek, and foods to avoid helpful in your journey to combat diabetes.

Exercise is a very beneficial complement to the ketogenic diet. The diet can be adapted to any exercise plan that you have and provides you with the best results when followed well. The aim is to ensure that the glucose that is needed for workouts is present in the body. With the proper planning of food intake and exercise, one would be able to mitigate the side effects—one such is the body shifting from its ketogenic state. Therefore, it is conceivable to be a weightlifter, a sportsperson, or anyone who desires to include exercise into their keto routine and still gain the rewards of the diet.

After reading this book, you have now a glimpse at the keto diet and have received enough information to aid you in making that decision to note that the diet will benefit your overall health and wellbeing and provide you with the quality of life you deserve. Whether through reading you have been convinced of applying this diet to your daily life or you were determined to do so before, this beginner's guide would have provided you with guidance, tips, tricks, and recipes that will allow you to implement it successfully.

The use of the keto diet in your life will extend beyond just weight loss and will help you to develop a better understanding of foods and allow you to be more aware of what you put into your body. If you do not take care of yourself, then who else will? Start the diet today and reap the benefits for you to live a long and happy life.